Penguin Books

Penguin Nursing Revision Notes
ORTHOPAEDIC NURSING

Other titles in this series:

Care for the Elderly
Ear, Nose and Throat Nursing
General Medical Nursing
Ophthalmic Nursing
Principles of Nursing
Surgical Nursing

Penguin Nursing Revision Notes
Advisory Editor: P. A. Downie

■ Orthopaedic Nursing

Revised edition

Penguin Books

PENGUIN BOOKS

Published by the Penguin Group
27 Wrights Lane, London W8 5TZ, England
Viking Penguin Inc., 40 West 23rd Street, New York, New York 10010, USA
Penguin Books Australia Ltd, Ringwood, Victoria, Australia
Penguin Books Canada Ltd, 2801 John Street, Markham, Ontario, Canada L3R 1B4
Penguin Books (NZ) Ltd, 182–190 Wairau Road, Auckland 10, New Zealand

Penguin Books Ltd, Registered Offices: Harmondsworth, Middlesex, England

First published 1983
This revised edition published in Penguin Books 1989
10 9 8 7 6 5 4 3 2 1

Copyright © Penguin Books Ltd, 1983, 1989
All rights reserved

Made and printed in Great Britain by
Cox and Wyman Ltd, Reading, Berks.
Typeset in 9/10½ pt Linotron 202 Galliard by
Rowland Phototypesetting Ltd, Bury St Edmunds, Suffolk

Except in the United States of America, this book is sold subject
to the condition that it shall not, by way of trade or otherwise, be lent,
re-sold, hired out, or otherwise circulated without the
publisher's prior consent in any form of binding or cover other than
that in which it is published and without a similar condition
including this condition being imposed on the subsequent purchaser

Contents

Advisory editor's note *vii*

1 General principles of orthopaedic nursing *1*

2 The principles of traction, splinting and management of plasters *8*

3 Fractures *19*

4 Spine and spinal injuries *41*

5 Joints *59*

6 Diseases affecting bone *78*

7 Conditions affecting children *93*

Advice for examination preparation *106*

Further reading *109*

Index *111*

Advisory editor's note

This series of revision aids first saw the light of day in the early 1980s and the books have been reprinted numerous times thus indicating that they fulfil a real need. Now they have been revised and updated. Many nurses, both tutors and ward sisters, have helped and advised in these revisions; they are too numerous to list individually but the warm thanks of the publishers and the advisory editor are extended to each of them.

These small books are not textbooks, *but* revision aids; consequently they aim to indicate principles and outlines rather than in-depth descriptions. Where specific treatments and care are discussed the reader should remember that they are not necessarily the only methods. All hospitals have their own laid-down treatment procedures and protocols and nurses must always apprise themselves of these.

Clinical terminology has been used throughout, though where there is an anatomical or scientific term this is shown also, and both terms are used simultaneously.

Care plans are shown in some of the books, but all the books lay emphasis on the four parts of the nursing process which can be turned into effective care plans, namely assessment, planning, implementation and evaluation. *Care* for patients is the *raison d'être* of all nursing and while these books are essentially revision aids for examinations, they nevertheless emphasize the nurse's role in the direct care of the patient.

Examinations might be described as 'necessary evils' in that they provide a means of ensuring that a person has reached an acceptable standard of competence. These books are intended as aids to help attain this standard; essentially they are for learners rather than nurses undergoing post-basic courses. Suggestions to help both study and the actual examination are included as is a short list of relevant reading. Specific references have not been included but learners are advised to make full use of their School of Nursing library and to seek help in learning how to seek out references from the librarian and their tutors.

In the 1850s, Florence Nightingale discussing how to teach nurses to nurse wrote in her *Notes on Nursing*: 'I do not pretend to teach her how, I ask her to teach herself, and for this purpose I venture to give her some hints'. Now, some hundred years on it falls to Penguin Books Limited to offer 'some hints' to the learner nurse of the present day as she prepares for her examinations.

P.D.
Norwich, 1988

1 General principles of orthopaedic nursing

The general principles of orthopaedic nursing are considered at the outset so that the learner can use them as a source of reference when applying them to the care of each patient.

■ ADMISSION

1 Planned/transfer
   a From the waiting list.
   b From another ward/hospital where specific treatment has begun.
2 Emergency from home or work
   a Via the GP or emergency services (sudden event).
   b Via the GP or consultant domiciliary visit following a period of illness at home.
   c Via the outpatient clinic (orthopaedic/fracture) which the patient has been attending.
   d Transfer from another ward/hospital where the patient was being treated for the same or different condition.

■ REASONS FOR ADMISSION

a The patient requires treatment which has to be carried out under continuous medical and nursing supervision.
b The patient has an acute condition which requires prompt medical intervention.
c To assess the extent of a disease process.
d For investigations to determine a diagnosis.

■ THE WARD ENVIRONMENT

The atmosphere on an orthopaedic ward is rather different to that of an acute general medical or surgical ward. The reasons include:

1 Patients are generally in for longer periods and get to know each other quite well.
2 For the same reason patients and those caring for them get to know each other well.
3 Often the long periods in hospital are for the immobilization of a part of the body so that patients themselves are not generally ill – or feeling constitutionally unwell for much of the time.

Ideally, orthopaedic wards should be spacious for the following reasons:

a Equipment used, e.g. balkan beams, traction, require more room.
b Some patients are in hospital for a long time and require room for their personal belongings.
c Because of splintage, crutches, wheelchairs, patients require room to manoeuvre when they are up and about.
d Nursing staff also require space around the bed area as several nurses are often required to lift and move a patient.
e Space is also required to facilitate the movement of beds from one part of the ward to another, e.g. to the treatment room for change of dressings, to the dayroom, or even outside, weather permitting.

Beds should have a hard base; alternatively, fracture boards will have to be used. Some beds may have an elevation device fitted on them; where these are not available, portable elevators or bed blocks may have to be used when required.

Generally speaking orthopaedic wards do not appear 'tidy' at a glance because of the various appliances, cradles, balkan beams, traction and so on, and beds are made to 'fit the patient', as it were. Uniform rows of neatly made beds is not usually the rule. Patient comfort and the practicalities of making the bed so as not to interfere with the function of the splintage or traction is the priority.

■ MEDICAL AND NURSING HISTORY AND PHYSICAL EXAMINATIONS

All patients admitted to an orthopaedic ward will undergo a full physical examination and have a clinical history taken by the doctor. The nurse will assess the patient and record her findings in the nursing care plan. The patient's condition and type of admission will determine the treatment and investigations which will follow. Some of the investigations will be routine, others will be specific; the doctor may also ask the nursing staff to carry out specific observations of the patient at regular intervals. The nurse should be familiar with what is routine, have a basic understanding of the specific investigations that may be required and of her responsibilities in relation to these investigations. Note will also be made of any drugs the patient may be taking; any drugs that the patient brings with him into hospital should be dealt with according to the hospital policy. The doctor will prescribe the drugs that the patient requires while in hospital which may or may not be the same as those which he was taking prior to the admission. Often at this point the doctor explains to the patient any treatment and investigations which may be necessary. The nature of impending surgery may be explained and discussed with the patient and the doctor will obtain the required consent.

The surgeon will need the patient's notes and radiographs. The nurse must ensure the patient's privacy and modesty by exposing only those parts required for examination. Both limbs are usually exposed for comparison. The surgeon will inspect any splints or shoes worn by the patient. He may wish to measure the length of a limb so that a tape measure should be readily available, and an angle measure (goniometer) may be required to measure the range of movement in the joints. A neurological examination tray should also be kept readily available. The patient may be examined standing and walking as well as lying in bed.

STRUCTURE AND FUNCTION

The learner should have some knowledge of the structure of the locomotor system, the range of movements of different parts of the body and normal body posture, both with regard to the patient and herself. The nurse caring for patients in any field must be able to demonstrate the ability to lift and move patients correctly without endangering herself or the patient. She must maintain the correct posture at all times. This is particularly important in orthopaedics as the patient's weight may be altered because of splintage, plaster and so on, so that more nurses may be required to lift such patients.

PSYCHOLOGICAL FACTORS

Admission into hospital can be a distressing experience for a patient. To be able to listen to patients and give them the opportunity to talk about their fears and anxieties is an important part of the nurse's function. She should be able to refer patients where necessary to people who are better able to help them cope with their problems. Maintaining good communication with patients and their families and keeping them informed of all relevant information at all times is also important.

Much fear and anxiety can be relieved at the time of admission if the patient and family are made to feel welcome. Following this initial meeting the relatives ought to be able to go home with ease of mind, knowing not only that the patient will be cared for by people who are concerned for him as a person, but also that information may be sought at any time.

■ SKIN AND HYGIENE

On admission and throughout his stay in hospital, observation should be made of the patient's skin colour, texture and cleanliness. The nurse should assess the patient's ability to perform his own personal hygiene and this will range from the patient's being able to care for himself without assistance, through the varying degrees of assistance to total dependency. Where relevant the use of the Norton or Waterlow scale to assess the risk of pressure sores developing may be helpful. Careful drying of the skin will help prevent soreness in those areas of the body that sweat. Special care of the skin will be required when the patient is pyrexial, with frequent washes, frequent changes of clothing, and use of cotton sheets and nightwear which are cooler for the patient. Special attention must be paid to those parts of the body which may be in a splint, with attention being given to both the splint itself as well as the skin. Splints can cause soreness of the skin if they do not fit properly.

The patient's hair must be kept clean and in good condition, the nails cleaned and manicured. Chiropody services are available to attend to the patient's feet and toenails as required, and the nurse must be aware of the importance of this expert foot care in certain conditions. Facilities should be available to maintain oral and dental care. Specific preparation of the skin may be required pre-operatively as requested by the surgeon. In the case of a limb, the surgeon usually marks the side requiring surgery, pre-operatively.

■ NUTRITION

The nurse should be able to assess the nutritional state of the patient and to report her observations to the medical staff. It may be that the patient is in a poor nutritional state for many reasons – psychological or socio-economic. The patient may require a special diet as part of the treatment as well as specific vitamins. It may also be necessary for the patient to eat his meals in positions that prove to be difficult at first and require perseverance and patience, e.g. the patient who has to maintain the supine position. It can be quite a frightening experience initially for a patient to have to eat his meals while on his back balancing the plate on his chest. The use of flexible straws facilitates drinking in this position. A head mirror will also be required.

For some hours postoperatively the patient's fluid and electrolyte balance may be maintained by intravenous infusion. While the doctor will set up the infusion and prescribe the fluid regime, it is the nurse's responsibility to ensure its working order, its maintenance and recording of the fluids. Pre-operatively food and fluids are withheld for up to six hours or as advised by the doctors, and the necessity for this is explained to the patient.

■ ELIMINATION

☐ *Bowels*

It is important to enquire of every patient the usual pattern of elimination, and to try to maintain this pattern. The nurse should recognize the need for privacy, the provision of facilities for hand washing following the use of bedpan/commode/sanichair, and to avoid the soiling of splints and plasters. The nurse should aim to prevent constipation; this is particularly important when the patient is relatively immobile.

☐ *Urine*

All patients admitted to the ward will have their urine tested routinely; urine may also have to be obtained for specific laboratory investigations. It should be observed that all patients pass urine within the first 24 hours of returning from theatre. Some patients, such as those who sustain injury to the spinal cord may require catheterization either continuously or intermittently and scrupulous cleanliness is required in subsequent care.

The use of appliances such as female urinals may be useful in some instances where the patient has to remain supine. Various other improvisations may also be needed. In any event complete privacy is essential to the patient for purposes of elimination.

■ OBSERVATIONS

A nurse may be asked to carry out general observations of the patient's appearance and specific observations such as the following:

a Temperature.
b Pulse (rate, rhythm, volume).
c Respirations (rate, depth, character).
d Blood pressure.
e Level of consciousness and response to stimuli.
f Peripheral pulses where appropriate.
g Observation of extremities: colour, temperature, sensitivity, movement.

The frequency with which these observations are recorded is determined by the patient's condition and his progress in response to therapy.

■ MOBILIZATION

The nurse should be able to assess the degree of mobility of each patient and decide how to help a patient with decreased mobility. Some movements may be undesirable, however, and have to be prevented. The nurse should have a basic understanding of types of surgery and of positions which the patient will have to avoid for a certain length of time. The physiotherapist plays an important role particularly with regard to specific exercises and ambulation of the patient. With regard to ambulation, maintenance of position, and mobilization of each individual patient the surgeon's instructions must be followed. In some instances the patient may be allowed up, without taking any weight on the affected limb (non-weight-bearing) – the patient must be made aware of this and be taught to use a walking aid or crutches. The patient should be moved correctly while in bed; the patient may require lifting as it may not be desirable to roll him from side to side. If the learner is not sure about the best way to move and turn a patient she should seek the help of senior colleagues. As the patient may be confined to bed for some time, regular change of position, or frequent relief of pressure is important in preventing pressure sores. Some patients may be able to assist with lifts if they are provided with suitable aids, e.g. 'monkey pole', others may require lifting by two or more nurses. Pillows should be placed to keep the patient in a good position in bed.

■ ADMINISTRATION OF DRUGS

Any drugs the patient may require are prescribed by the doctor and administered accordingly. They may include analgesics, antibiotics, vitamins, anti-inflammatory drugs and steroids for certain conditions.

INVESTIGATIONS

Specific investigations will be discussed in the relevant chapters. The nurse must be aware of her responsibilities in managing the patient, before, during and after each procedure.

REHABILITATION

The rehabilitation that patients require varies considerably. Each patient should be assessed at the outset and continuously in relation to the amount and type of help and advice they may require before their discharge home. The physiotherapist, occupational therapist, medical social worker, disablement resettlement officer, dietician, and others, all have important roles to play in a patient's rehabilitation.

2 The principles of traction, splinting and management of plasters

This chapter indicates:
1 The most usually encountered types of traction and the management of the patient on traction.
2 The observations that should be made when a splint is being used.
3 The nursing management of a patient with a plaster cast.

Traction can be described as a force or a pull which is applied to a part of the body. It may be used for:
a Immobilization following fractures thereby maintaining reduction for a prescribed period.
b Correcting some deformities, e.g. scoliosis.
c Securing the immobilization of an inflamed joint, e.g. rheumatoid arthritis.

■ TYPES OF TRACTION

■ Fixed traction

An example is to be seen in the force exerted between two fixed points of a Thomas' bed splint (Fig. 1).

■ Balanced traction

This is achieved by a force applied by weights and pulleys. The counter traction is achieved by the patient's body when the foot of the bed is elevated. An example of this is Hamilton Russell traction (Fig. 2).

A combination of fixed and balanced traction may also be employed. By application of a Thomas' splint and further suspension of this on weights and pulleys a combination is achieved which facilitates greater movement for the patient in bed, without interfering with the immobilization of the affected part. This is sometimes known as *sliding traction*.

There are several of these types of traction which can be modified to suit individual patients without deviating from the principles of traction.

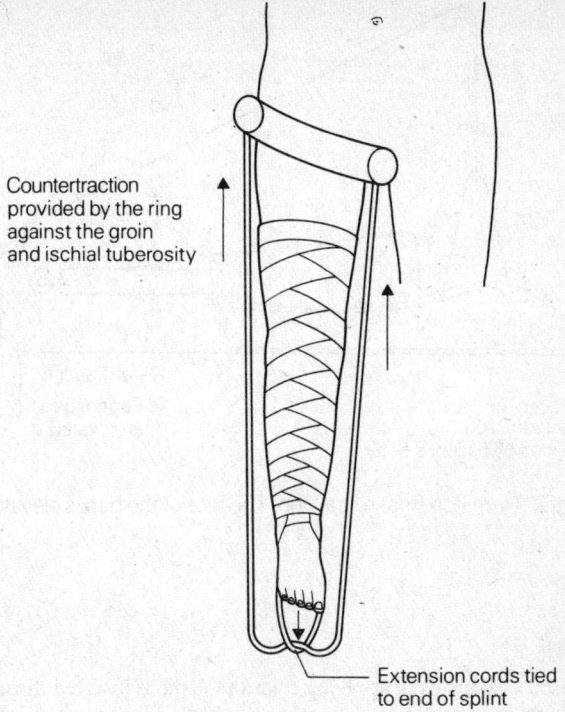

Fig. 1 Thomas' bed splint

■ METHODS USED FOR THE APPLICATION OF TRACTION

■ Skin

Extension strapping is applied to the skin which is used as a means of applying the force. Skin extensions may be adhesive or non-adhesive. If the skin extensions are zinc adhesive, the skin should first be shaved and then painted with tincture of benzoin (Friar's Balsam). This will prevent the skin's reacting to the zinc adhesive plaster.

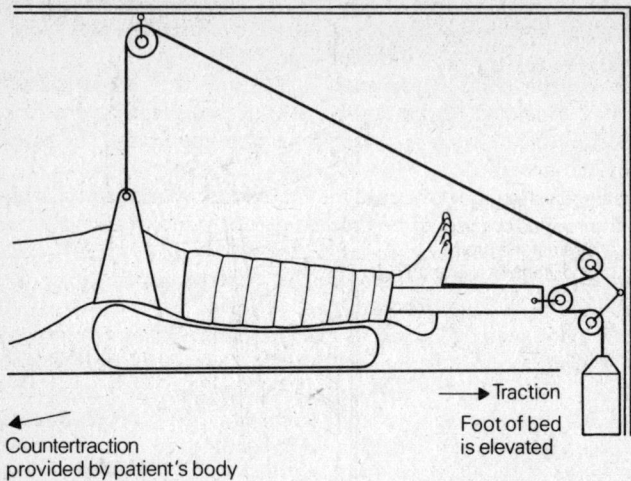

Fig. 2 Hamilton Russell traction. The foot of the bed is elevated

■ Skeletal

Bone is used as a means of applying traction. A pin is inserted through the bone, which is attached to a stirrup to which is attached weights and pulleys. Pins used may be:
a Denham's pin
b Steinmann's pin
c Kirschner wire.
More weight can be used with this type of traction.

■ NURSING OBSERVATIONS OF PATIENTS ON TRACTION

■ Skin traction

a The traction should be maintained at all times, unless otherwise indicated by the surgeon. In the event that weights are removed it is usual to apply temporary traction which may be applied manually.
b The skin must be observed regularly to ensure there are no breaks or

irritations developing. It is usual to remove the bandages daily and observe the extensions at the same time.
c Check all the bony prominences and ensure they are well padded. Padding should be placed under the knee to prevent hyperextension. Inspection of the heels and patella are also important. The patella is often left uncovered.
d Extremities should be observed for warmth, movement and sensitivity.
e Cords and pulleys should be checked regularly and weights allowed to hang freely, not touching the bed or floor.
f Encourage the patient to practise the exercises (isometric or active) which he will be taught by the physiotherapist.
g Patients may sometimes complain of discomfort following the application of skin traction, due to perspiration of the limb or limbs, the growth of hair which was previously removed for the application of skin extensions of the adhesive type, and other possible reactions. No complaint made by the patient should go unnoticed.
h Note changes in limb alignment – e.g. drop foot, external rotation. Any abnormalities should be promptly reported.

■ Skeletal traction

The points about the management of cords, weights and pulleys and the maintenance of traction apply also to skeletal traction. In addition the following observations are made.
a The pin sites at the point of entry through the skin must be kept clean, and may be covered with a key-hole dressing. Any discharge from these areas must be reported.
b Corks are placed on the exposed tips of the pins to avoid cutting the patient and those caring for him.
c It is important to ensure that movement of the pin in its tract does not occur, as this may give rise to infection.
d Bony prominences are checked.

■ GENERAL NURSING POINTS FOR CONSIDERATION

Patients on traction may, rarely, have to lie flat (supine) continuously. Where this is the case consideration will have to be given to things like the position of the patient's locker, help with feeding, cutting up food, and use of feeders/flexible straws. A head mirror is necessary. Mostly, however, patients on traction are encouraged to move within their limitations and to become independent.

The bedclothes should not inhibit the effect of the traction in any way, but should serve to keep the patient warm and comfortable. The limb in traction may be kept warm by a small separate blanket.

Care must be maintained of the patient's back, with an adequate number of nurses to lift the patient slightly at frequent intervals to relieve pressure. If the patient is able he should be taut to raise himself by pulling on the overhead monkey pole. The bottom sheet and draw sheet must be kept taut, crease and crumb free. The bony prominences and skin on the back and buttocks must be inspected regularly.

Patients may experience some difficulty using bedpans. Patients should be placed on bedpans and pillows arranged so that adequate support is provided for the patient's body. It also avoids further discomfort for the patient to ensure that the usual pattern of bowel action is maintained so that constipation may be avoided. Suppositories and, or, enemas may have to be administered if this occurs, further distressing the patient. A well-balanced diet, adequate fluid intake and possibly a mild aperient as prescribed will help prevent the development of constipation. To avoid the development of renal calculi as a result of immobilization adequate fluid intake is important.

The patient should be told about the purpose of the traction and the importance of maintaining the correct position while on it.

The patient may be on traction for a number of weeks and every effort must be made to prevent boredom, although there will be times when the patient feels frustrated and should be allowed to talk through his feelings. Family and friends should be encouraged to visit and if they can arrange to spread their visits so that not everyone arrives at the same time, this will help to break up the day for the patient. The occupational therapist may be able to give suitable advice.

At all times the nurse must ensure that the traction remains functional. Any complaints made by the patient *must* be reported to the surgeon.

■ SPLINTS

Splints are used for a variety of reasons including immobilization of a part; to correct deformity; to maintain the affected part in corrected position; and to provide traction as in the Thomas' bed splint; calipers can be used to relieve weight. *Night* splints may be used to rest joints and to maintain a functional position. It is beyond the scope of this text to describe every

type of splint, and information regarding them can be found in appropriate textbooks. The nurse should consider the following points about splints.
a To serve their purpose splints should fit correctly.
b Incorrectly fitting splints can give rise to pressure/plaster sores.
c The splint itself should be looked after and kept in good condition.
d The skin underneath the splint requires careful inspection. Bony prominences and areas subjected to pressure must be closely observed. The skin must be kept clean and dry.
e Observation of extremities, including swelling, circulation, warmth, sensitivity, movement, must be scrupulously maintained.

Should a sore develop the cause must be found and removed and dressings applied to the sore. Any leather material on splints must be kept in good condition to avoid cracking.

Thomas' bed splint. Particular mention is made of this splint as it is frequently encountered. Special attention must be paid to the ring area. Initially, the skin beneath the ring should be gently moved at frequent intervals – later the intervals can be increased and the patient taught to do this himself. Provided the ring fits correctly there should be no undue pressure in the groin or on the ischial tuberosity.

■ PLASTER CASTS/SPLINTS

Plaster of Paris as a means of immobilization has been used for many years and is effective. Recent years have seen the development of plaster which can be immersed in water (Hexcelite) and is lighter in weight. There are other materials also available but these will not be considered. This discussion relates to the management of the conventional plaster of Paris. The nurse should, during the trauma and orthopaedic module, familiarize herself with the common plaster room instruments, so that she is aware of their functions and, if possible, observe the application of plaster of Paris.

■ Points to remember when caring for a patient while plaster is drying

1 The plaster cast should be placed on a pillow/pillows covered with a waterproof material.
2 Whenever the patient is lifted the cast should be supported in its entirety and handled with the palms of the hands so that fingertips do not cause indentation of the plaster.

3 During drying the plaster should not be covered, but allowed to dry at room temperature. Artificial heat should not be applied. If plasters cover a large area such as spicas the patient will require turning regularly in one piece to facilitate drying.
4 In the case of a limb the extremities require observation – circulation, temperature, movement and sensitivity.
5 Postoperatively any bleeding which soaks into the plaster is monitored by outlining the stain with a marking pen. An assessment can then be made as to whether blood loss is continuing.
6 The cast should be checked for cracks and indentations to make sure that the edges are not causing pressure on the patient's skin.
7 Vital observations may be necessary following the application of a cast, e.g. blood pressure, pulse, etc.
8 When the patient is lifted on to a bedpan, careful use and arrangement of pillows will ensure that the cast (as well as the patient) is adequately supported. Care must be taken not to soil the cast with urine or faeces.
9 Joints not encased in plaster must be exercised.

■ Further management of plasters

The patient and the plaster cast must be continuously observed and the nurse must bear in mind the possibilities of a plaster sore. The patient may complain of any of the following which may indicate a sore:
1 A burning sensation or pain beneath the plaster.
2 *a* Restlessness during the night.
   b Children may be fretful.
3 Itching beneath the cast.

The nurse may observe the following:
1 A rise in body temperature – (local heat may be felt over the cast).
2 A distinct and offensive odour.
3 The presence of a discharge.

Should a sore develop a window is generally cut in the cast so that the sore may be dressed aseptically.

In some instances, particularly following recent trauma or surgery, the plaster may need to be split. If the nurse is in any doubt about the circulation, sensation, mobility, warmth of the extremities, she *must* report it without any delay.

■ SCOTCH CAST AND DELTA LITE CAST

These casts are made from synthetic materials and are lightweight, porous and able to breathe. A major advantage to these casts is that the patient can be weight-bearing in half an hour after application.

Like plaster of Paris casts the Scotch Cast and the Delta Lite ones take a while to get used to.

■ Special drying instructions

The cast can be kept clean by wiping it with a damp cloth. Soap is not recommended.

If the cast becomes accidentally wet it will not break down, but it is essential that the correct drying procedure is carried out:

1 Remove excess water; this can be done by wrapping the cast in a towel and also by resting the cast on a pad of towels.
2 Use a blow-type hairdrier on the wet cast until the padding under the cast has dried out. It is important that the padding is completely dry because dampness under the cast can cause a skin irritation.

■ GENERAL CAST CARE FOR THE PATIENT

1 Follow any instructions carefully regarding physical activity.
2 If a cast needs support and you have to use furniture, put a pillow or a towel next to the surface to avoid scratching the furniture.
3 It is advisable not to trim or cut down the length of the cast yourself as you may prolong healing.
4 Avoid inserting instruments into the cast for scratching as you may damage the skin and cause a serious infection.

■ WHEN TO SEEK HELP

1 If you have constant pain and the medication your doctor has given you is not effective.
2 If and when your cast feels too loose or too tight.
3 If your cast cracks or becomes broken.
4 If pressure develops beneath the cast or if your cast is rubbing and it becomes painful.
5 If you notice whitish or bluish discolouration at the distal end of the

limb within the cast. You may experience pins and needles at the same time.
6 If you experience continual coldness of the limb/cast.

■ PRACTICE QUESTIONS

1 *What is meant by the following terms?*
   a Fixed traction
   b Balanced traction
   c Skeletal traction
   d Skin traction
   e Plaster of Paris
   f Plaster sore
   g Hyperextension
   h Isometric exercises (static)
   i Splints
   j Alignment.
2 *Briefly explain the following*
   a Why may traction be applied by the skeletal method in preference to that of the skin?
   b What preparation would the patient's limb/limbs require prior to the application of skin extension?
   c Why is it necessary for a patient whose limbs are in traction to be aware that he should maintain the correct position of the rest of his body?
   d Why is it important for splints to fit correctly?
   e Why is it important to check the circulation, movement, sensation and temperature of the extremities when a limb is immobilized in a form of splintage?
   f Explain what is meant by a plaster cast that is bivalved.
   g Why does a plaster cast require handling by the palms and to be moved in its entirety while drying?
   h What factors may contribute to the development of a plaster sore?
3 *Mark the following statements True or False*
   a Drop foot may develop from pressure on the common peroneal nerve.
   b Immobilization can cause increased calcium in the blood due to decalcification of bones.
   c Plaster sores develop only if the plaster has been incorrectly applied.
   d An offensive odour can be the first sign of a plaster sore.

e If a deep sore has developed beneath the plaster the patient may no longer complain of pain.
f Following the removal of a plaster cast the patient's limb will usually require washing in warm soapy water to remove dead skin that has collected.
g A plaster is *never* removed altogether without first consulting the surgeon.
h It is frequently necessary, indeed desirable, to wash the patient's skin underneath the ring of the Thomas' bed splint.
i It is not necessary to check the knots and traction cord once the traction has been set in position.

■ Answers

1 *a* A pull or a force achieved between two fixed points.
  b A pull or a force is applied by the use of weights and pulleys and counter-traction is applied by the patient's body pulling in the other direction, the latter being effectively achieved by elevating the end of the bed accommodating the weights.
  c A method of applying traction directly through a bone.
  d When the skin is used as a means of applying the traction.
  e A substance impregnated into bandages which are soaked, applied to a limb and form a hard and effective form of splintage.
  f A sore which may develop on the skin which is encased in a plaster cast.
  g A joint which is in a position of extension becomes over extended.
  h Exercising the muscles without actually moving the limb.
  i An appliance which may be applied to a part of the body to maintain that part in the desired position.
  j Alignment is a term used to describe the correct position of one part in relation to another. One can talk about body alignment – when one part of the body is in alignment with the other; or perhaps in the case of a fracture that the two bone ends are in the correct position in relation to one another – in alignment.

2 *a* Skeletal traction once applied, surprisingly enough, is often more comfortable to the patient and has the advantage of allowing more weights to be applied. It is used mainly in the treatment of fractures.
  b If non-adhesive extensions are used the skin requires no preparation. If the adhesive-type extensions are used (they are supplied commercially) the skin should be inspected for abrasions and may require shaving. Tincture of benzoin is applied to the skin so that the extensions adhere more effectively and protect the skin, unless its use is contra-indicated by the manufacturers.

18 Orthopaedic Nursing

   c So that the patient's body remains in alignment, and does not distort the function of the traction.
   d If they do not fit correctly they are probably not fulfilling their function and they could also cause the formation of splint sores.
   e To ensure that the splintage is not interfering with the nerve and circulatory supply to the limb.
   f A cast which is cut along its length in two places so that one half may be removed.
   g If the fingers are used they can cause indentations in the plaster giving rise to sores later; if the plaster is not supported in its entirety it may crack.
   h
- Cracks, cutting into the skin.
- A plaster which is loose.
- A plaster which is incorrectly applied.
- Inadequate padding of bony prominences.
- Foreign bodies which find their way inside the cast, e.g. crumbs, beads, etc.
- Incorrect handling during drying.

3 *a* True
  b True
  c False
  d True
  e True
  f True
  g True
  h False
  i False.

3 Fractures

The objectives of this chapter are to:
1 Describe the structure of bone and the functions of the skeleton.
2 Describe the sequence of events that take place in the process of bone healing.
3 Classify fractures according to types.
4 List common fractures of the upper limbs.
5 List common fractures of the lower limbs.
6 Describe the management of a patient with a fractured pelvis.
7 State the principles of management and care of a patient with fractures.

■ STRUCTURE OF BONE

Although bone is a hard solid structure, it is living connective tissue requiring oxygen and nutrients.

The bone cell is called the osteocyte. Microscopically the bone cells are arranged in small depressions called lacunae surrounded by intercellular collagenous substance in which the calcium salts are stored. Within the intercellular substance are many tiny channels (canaliculi) which serve to connect the lacunae thereby supplying the osteocytes with oxygen and nutrients.

Bone is of two types:
a *Cancellous bone* (spongy) in which is found the red bone marrow. It is found in the ends of long bones and flat bones such as the skull, sternum and ribs. It is here that blood cells are formed from the haemocytoblasts. The arrangement of red bone marrow in babies and infants is slightly different. Cancellous bone appears to the naked eye like a sponge – visually but not in texture. The spaces in between the thin bands of interwoven bones are quite open compared to the second type of bone called the compact bone.
b *Compact bone* is dense and very solid and found on the outer aspect of the bone. The cells of compact bone receive their vital supplies through the organized series of interconnecting channels called the Haversian system.

Bones are covered by a tough fibrous tissue – the periosteum. The innermost layer of periosteum consists of osteoblasts which are active bone-forming cells which enhance the growth and repair process of bone. Other cells found in bone which are of importance are the osteoclasts, these play a part in the re-absorption of bone tissue thereby giving the bone its desired shape.

The parts of bones which join together to form a joint are usually covered with cartilage (articular or hyaline cartilage).

Figure 3 shows the structure of a typical long bone. In the centre along the length of a long bone is a hollow cavity called the medullary cavity which contains yellow bone marrow.

Bones are generally classified according to their shape:
i Long bones, e.g. bones of the limbs such as the femur.
ii Flat bones, e.g. scapula.

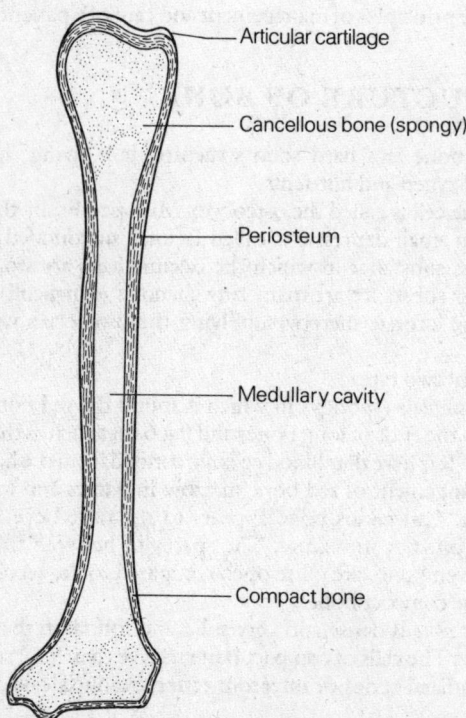

Fig. 3 The internal structure of a long bone

iii Short bones, often small and cuboid in shape, such as those of the wrist (carpal bones).
iv Irregular bones are those that do not fall into the above categories and as the term suggests are of many different shapes, e.g. vertebrae.
v Sesamoid bone describes one which has developed in a tendon, e.g. patella.

■ THE FUNCTIONS OF THE SKELETON

1 To provide support for the soft tissue structures of the body and to protect organs, e.g. lungs, brain.
2 To store calcium for the body's needs. (It is the deposition of calcium and minerals that give bone its strength.)
3 The formation of blood cells in the red bone marrow.
4 Bones provide a means for the attachment of muscles. (Muscles are attached to bones by tendons.)
5 Bones provide a form of leverage when one part of the body is moved in relation to another by the muscles.
6 Superficial bones can be used to locate various other structures in the body by virtue of the fact that they are so easily felt.

■ THE HEALING OF BONE (Fig. 4)

Healing of bone takes place in five stages. When a fracture occurs the vessels of the Haversian system are torn so that bleeding takes place at the fracture site, thereby forming a clot (Stage 1). The periosteum is also torn depriving the fragments of their blood supply.

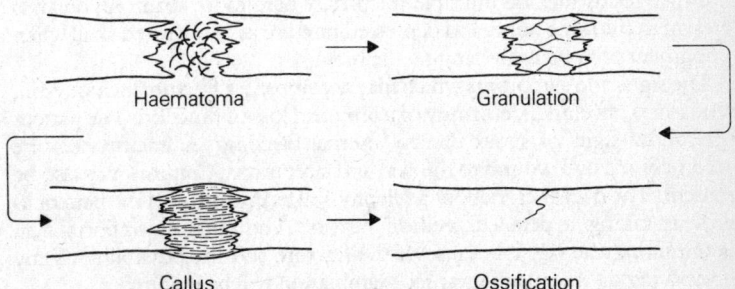

Fig. 4 Repair of a fracture

Various cells then come into play, particularly the osteoblasts of the periosteum, to provide a bridging structure at the fracture site in order to enhance union of the bone by means of callus formation (Stages 2 and 3).

New capillaries and cells with bone-forming properties lay down a network of thin strips of bone and replace the fragments deprived of blood (Stage 4). With callus formation and union the fracture site is then refashioned so that the correct relationship of compact bone and a central cavity is achieved (Stage 5).

■ CLASSIFICATION OF FRACTURES (Fig. 5)

Fractures are classified usually according to the line of fracture. It must be remembered that although a fracture is referred to as the loss of continuity in a bone, i.e. a break, there is also some damage to the surrounding soft tissue structure, e.g. muscles.

Fractures without the presence of a wound are said to be simple or closed fractures; fractures may be caused by either direct violence (when the fracture occurs directly beneath the site of impact) or indirect violence where a fracture occurs in a bone other than that directly beneath the site of impact.

Depending on the site, the fragment of a fractured bone may penetrate an organ or damage nerves and blood vessels; these fractures are then called complicated fractures. Sometimes, when a bone is fractured, the overlying skin may also be damaged giving rise to what is termed a compound fracture. This does not necessarily mean the bone fragments have to be protruding through the skin, but that there is contact between the fracture site and the surrounding environment. The risks of infection are therefore a potential hazard.

Other terms include multiple fracture, where more than one break is present in the same bone, and depressed fracture as in fractured skull when a fragment of bone is pressing on the brain.

The signs and symptoms which may accompany a fracture include pain, tenderness, swelling, deformity of a limb and loss of function. The patient may show signs of shock due to internal bleeding. A fracture may be accompanied by a wound to the skin and lacerations. Crepitus may also be present. The doctor carries out a full physical examination of the patient as well as taking a detailed medical history. The latter is important in determining the possible cause of the fracture and the possibility of any underlying disease. Radiographic examination will be required.

(a) Transverse fracture

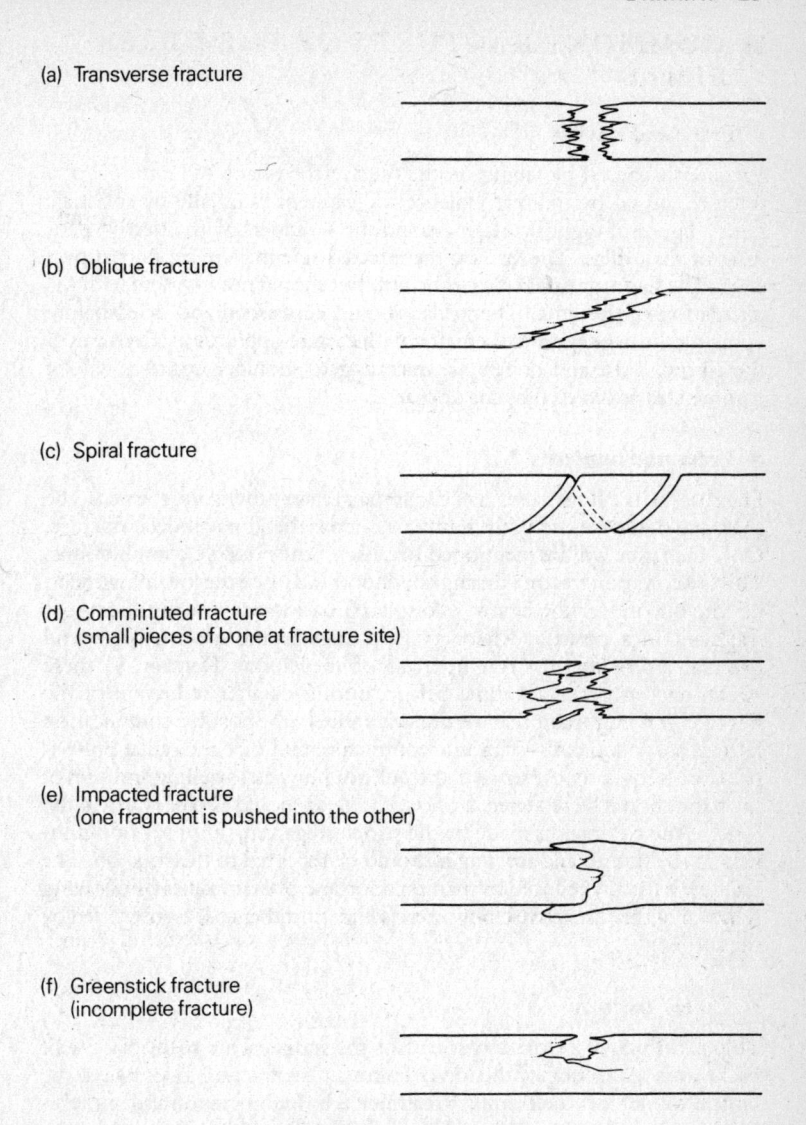

(b) Oblique fracture

(c) Spiral fracture

(d) Comminuted fracture
    (small pieces of bone at fracture site)

(e) Impacted fracture
    (one fragment is pushed into the other)

(f) Greenstick fracture
    (incomplete fracture)

Fig. 5 Types of fracture

COMMON FRACTURES OF THE UPPER LIMBS

Fractured clavicle

Frequently caused by falling on the outstretched hand (an example of a fracture caused by indirect violence). Treatment is usually by splintage with a figure-of-eight bandage around the shoulders, with effective padding of the axillae. The arm on the affected side may be supported by a sling. The bandage applied must be firm but should not interfere with the circulation of the limb. The axillae should be washed and dried before applying the bandage and thereafter with each re-application. Exercises of the elbow, wrist and fingers are encouraged, shoulder exercises will be commenced as directed by the doctor.

Fractured humerus

Fractures of the humerus can occur at the greater tuberosity, the neck, the shaft and the lower end of the humerus, such as the supracondylar fracture. Only the latter will be mentioned because of the possible complications. This is a common fracture during childhood and often the lower fragment, i.e. the one nearer the elbow, is displaced backwards, leaving the upper fragment in a position where it could damage the median nerve and brachial artery as they run in front of the elbow. Damage to these structures can occur any time before, during or after reduction of the fracture. It is important that the nurse is aware of the possible complication known as Volkmann's ischaemic contracture and that the radial pulse is palpated frequently. Absence of the pulse or blueness, swelling and pain of the hand should be reported at once. The hand should also be warm to the touch. Any complaints made by the patient regarding a feeling of numbness in the thumb and forefinger should be reported to the surgeon. The fracture is usually reduced by manipulation and plaster fixation. Following removal of the cast active elbow exercises are commenced, as instructed by the surgeon.

Colles' fracture

This is a fracture of the lower end of the radius. Due to displacement backwards and tilting of the lower fragment the fracture gives rise to the typical 'dinner fork' deformity. Treatment is by manipulation and immobilization in a plaster cast extending from the knuckles to just below the elbow joint. The thumb and fingers remain free, and they, as well as the elbow and shoulder joints, are exercised. A sling may be used for the first few days until the swelling subsides. The cast may be removed after about five weeks and full use of the limb is encouraged.

Any rings on the fingers should be removed in case swelling develops, making their removal difficult.

■ FRACTURES OF THE LOWER LIMBS

■ The femur

The femur is the large thigh bone. The head of the femur articulates with the acetabulum of the hip bone, and the lower end articulates with the tibia (the knee joint). Between the shaft and the femoral head is the neck of femur, which is a common site of fracture particularly in elderly women.

The femur is well covered by muscles – the quadriceps anteriorly and the hamstrings posteriorly.

Fractures of the neck of femur are divided into those that occur within the capsule, i.e. intracapsular (these fractures can often interfere with the blood supply to the femoral head); and extracapsular fractures which are found in the trochanteric region, and do not generally interfere with the supply of blood to the head of the femur.

The treatment selected depends on the age of the patient and type of fracture. As elderly patients are more susceptible to the complications of bed rest operative measures may be considered as they will usually allow earlier mobilization. Intracapsular fractures, because of the possible interference with the blood supply with subsequent necrosis of the head of femur, may be treated by replacement of the femoral head with a prosthesis, e.g. Austin Moore or Thompson (see p. 71). Extracapsular fractures may be treated surgically by the insertion of pins or nail-plate. Splintage or traction may be required pre-operatively. Alternatively the fracture may be treated conservatively by means of balanced traction. Some surgeons favour applying the traction using the skeletal method as it is more comfortable for the patient. (A plaster cast may also be applied to incorporate the pin which is inserted into the tibial tubercle.) Others may use skin extensions for the application of traction which is usually the Hamilton Russell type. Once traction is established the degree of abduction ordered by the surgeon *has* to be maintained, as well as preventing external rotation of the limb.

Because these types of fracture are commonly seen in the elderly and thus frequently encountered in the trauma and orthopaedic units of general hospitals, let us consider the nursing management together with the social implications surrounding the management of elderly patients.

NURSING CARE OF THE ELDERLY ORTHOPAEDIC PATIENT

Position of the patient in the ward and position in bed

When the patient is first admitted to the ward he will be placed in an area where he can be continuously observed, as he may be in a state of shock as well as in pain. It may also be of comfort to the patient to be able to see nurses most of the time, as some elderly patients may not have been in hospital for many years or, occasionally, never before, in which case it will be quite a daunting experience. Consideration must also be given to the fact that elderly patients may become confused with the strange clinical environment of the hospital.

The patient's position in bed is usually semi-recumbent supported with pillows and a backrest. A cradle is placed in the bed to avoid the weight of the bed clothes resting on the affected limb. The affected limb may be placed on a pillow – lengthwise – so that the heel is kept off the bed. (Sandbags may be placed on either side of the affected limb to immobilize it.) Traction may be ordered temporarily, or arrangements will be made to prepare the patient for theatre at the outset. If the patient is confused cot sides (sometimes called safety sides) may be necessary.

Assessment

The usual admission records are completed and an initial assessment of the patient is made which will then continue throughout his stay in hospital. It is important to establish whether or not the patient has living relatives, how available they are, how closely related and how much support they will be able to offer the patient during hospitalization and on return home. The discharge of the patient should be considered from the outset. It has to be remembered that many of these patients are well into their eighties and that those relatives who feel responsible for them are themselves in their sixties. The type of house that the person lives in is of considerable importance, whether or not they have a toilet which is easily accessible, the possibilities of having a bed brought downstairs on return home and so on; such questions must be taken into account. Once settled in the hospital with treatment prescribed by the surgeon all of the above can be discussed with the family and caring team.

Teamwork in this instance is of paramount importance and the medical social worker should be called in at the earliest opportunity. Sometimes patients have no living relatives by the time they themselves have reached the eighties, but it would be wrong to assume that it is only those who are alone who will require the services that are available to the elderly when they are discharged home. Each person has to be assessed individually, Some patients make such a recovery that they are able to return to their homes with the minimum of help, others will require a great deal of help, others unfortunately may not be able to return to their own homes at all and may require accommodation where a certain amount of supervision is provided.

■ Skin and general hygiene

When surgery is decided upon the affected limb may require shaving and washing with soap and water. If the surgeon favours the use of special antiseptic preparation then this should be done.

An assessment should be made of the general condition of the patient's skin at the outset. Bruising on the affected side should be noted, and any other damage to the skin which may have been incurred during the time of injury. The condition of the patient's skin may be an indication of how the patient has been able to care for himself up to the time of injury. The patient's usual routine regarding bathing should be established so that when he is allowed up, his usual pattern can be maintained; until such time, however, the patient will be bathed in bed, and encouraged from the outset to wash as much of himself as he can manage. The back, buttocks and lower limbs will be done by the nurses. Frequent observations of the skin for red marks from pressure must be made. It is perhaps a mistake to assume that the elderly aren't so particular about their appearance as the younger generation, so washing the hair and styling it to the patient's liking will also be of benefit. In some hospitals hairdressers are available for this purpose. Nails should be kept clean and short and the patient encouraged to manicure them himself. It may be necessary to remove any nail polish and *not* allow it to be replaced. This is to enable the doctor/nurse to observe the colour of the nail or any change in it. Toenails also should be kept clean and short and cut correctly. If the patient is a diabetic, care of the feet and toenails should be done by the chiropodist. The patient may well have dentures and should be encouraged to clean them in the way he usually does either by brushing or soaking them in a solution – (perhaps overnight) – and facilities should be provided so that the patient can continue to care for dentures himself.

■ Eating and drinking

If the patient requires surgical treatment food and drink will be withheld for up to six hours prior to surgery. The necessity for this should be explained to the patient. If the patient is in a poor nutritional state prior to surgery this may require correction beforehand. Otherwise the patient should be offered a balanced diet and the nurse should be able to anticipate the amount of help required by the patient so that the meal can be eaten with ease and comfort. Cutting up the meat, for instance, and ensuring that utensils are within reach of the patient. Protection should be afforded so that the patient does not feel anxious about soiling the linen. He should acquire as much independence as possible in eating meals, but initially some help may be required and if appetite is poor the diet can be supplemented by nutritional drinks.

Postoperatively the fluid balance may be maintained by an intravenous infusion, but the patient must be encouraged to take oral fluids and diet as soon as he is able to tolerate them.

A dental surgeon may need to be consulted if the patient is unable to take his diet because of dentures that do not fit properly or perhaps because the patient has no dentures at all.

Roughage may have to be included in the diet so that constipation may be avoided. Fluids should also be given regularly and help may be required in pouring drinks and making sure that the patient is able to manipulate and reach the tumbler. Time and encouragement may be required in ensuring that the patient actually drinks the fluid – this is important as elderly patients can quickly become dehydrated. A strict fluid balance chart should be kept.

■ Elimination

□ Urine

The urine is tested when the patient is first admitted into hospital. Until the patient is allowed up a bedpan (or slipper pan) will be used. Sensible use of pillows to support the patient while on the bedpan, particularly the 'small of the back', will do much to alleviate a situation which is all too often strenuous and uncomfortable. As soon as the patient is able, a monkey pole should be provided so that he can lift himself off the bed to accommodate the positioning of the bedpan. Note is made of the urinary output and occasionally catheterization may be necessary; however a pattern of micturition is established as soon as possible.

If the patient is incontinent an attempt is made to assess the patient's pattern of elimination, by recording how often the patient is incontinent and therefore offering the patient a bedpan at the appropriate times. A specimen of urine may be obtained for culture and sensitivity if it is suspected the incontinence is due to a urinary infection. As the patient progresses and when the surgeon allows, use can be made of the commode and toilet.

☐ *Bowels*

Prevention of constipation is important. This is achieved by adequate roughage in the diet and plenty of fluids. It is also necessary to establish with the patient at the outset his normal bowel habits as the pattern of emptying the bowel varies from one person to another. As far as is possible his own individual pattern should be maintained. Some elderly patients may have been taking mild forms of medication for purposes of maintaining a daily bowel action for years and the doctor may allow its continued use by prescribing it for the patient. It should always be remembered that constipation, in the elderly in particular, can give rise to the complication of faecal impaction with subsequent partial or complete obstruction. Furthermore, constipation may lead to mental confusion in the elderly. The patient initially may require help with cleaning himself following the use of a bedpan.

■ **Mobility**

In orthopaedics mobility assumes the utmost importance. It may seem somewhat confusing to the learner that patients start mobilizing at different time intervals postoperatively or following certain types of conservative treatments. It cannot be overemphasized that getting a patient up and mobile must be in accordance with the surgeon's wishes. There are no hard and fast rules and mobilizing is according to the disease process and specific treatment. For example, replacement of the femoral head with a prosthesis may or may not be followed by a period of immobilization on Hamilton–Russell traction.

The patient's position in bed must be changed regularly or pressure must be otherwise relieved. When the patient is in the semi-recumbent position much weight is taken on the sacral area. When possible the patient should be encouraged to lift himself slightly off the bed at frequent intervals with the use of a monkey pole. The patient may also flex the knee of the unaffected limb and with the arms firmly placed on the mattress can ease the buttocks off the bed. Slight movements from side to side may be permissible but care must be taken in maintaining the position of the affected limb. Special attention should be paid to the heels – the leg on the affected side may be supported on a pillow so that the heel is clear of the bed. While careful selection of appropriate aids helps in the prevention of sores they are not substitutes for nurses' frequently observing those areas which are particularly susceptible. Sitting the patient completely upright in bed is generally avoided so that the hips are not flexed, particularly following replacement of the femoral head as this may cause the prosthesis to dislocate.

Physiotherapy is given in the form of breathing exercises, movements of the feet and toes and general strengthening exercises. The nurse will be shown how she may encourage the patient to practise the exercises regularly. The physiotherapist will be responsible for getting the patient out of bed and for advising the nursing staff about the most appropriate walking aids. The occupational therapist assesses the patient for any aids he may require to help him with dressing and what household jobs the patient is capable of doing before he goes home. The nurses can also encourage the patient to carry out activities in the ward when he has reached the stage to do so. To encourage the patient to do things for himself will enable an acceptable level of independence to be achieved. To perform tasks for the patient which he is able to do for himself – often because it's quicker – is in the long term to do the patient a disservice.

When the patient starts to get out of bed, variable height beds are ideal. Once the patient is mobile he can get dressed in his own clothes and be encouraged to walk about. It should be remembered that sitting in a chair for long periods can give rise to pressure sores developing.

■ Rest and sleep

Rest and adequate sleep can be best achieved by discovering at the outset what was the patient's usual kind of day. What time does he usually retire at night, does he usually sleep all night? Some elderly people get up at a regular time to make themselves a drink. Does the patient have a particular drink or nightcap he likes to have prior to going to sleep, and so on; as far as possible these habits should be maintained: night sedation should be avoided for elderly patients because they tend not to tolerate it well and may sleep well into the next day, disrupting their usual pattern. Every effort should be made to find out why a patient may be having difficulty in sleeping.

■ Communication

There must be good communication between all the disciplines caring for the patient.

The patient should be kept aware of his progress and adequate explanations given regarding the importance of maintaining certain positions and so on, so that the patient is involved fully with his treatment and care.

Relatives must be kept fully informed and involved with discharge preparations.

■ FRACTURED SHAFT OF FEMUR

A fractured shaft of femur can be treated surgically by means of a Küntscher intramedullary nail, plate and screws, or bone grafting. Alternatively, reduction of the fracture may be achieved by manipulation and immobilization in a Thomas' bed splint. The patient is measured correctly for a Thomas' splint. The surgeon reduces the fracture under a local or general anaesthetic, skin extensions are applied to the limb, followed by application of the splint already prepared with slings. The extension cords are then pulled taut and tied to the end of the splint (fixed traction). The whole splint can be suspended by the use of weights and pulleys. Balanced traction can also be used by means of a skeletal pin and suspension of the splint, allowing movement of the patient in bed without interfering with the reduced fracture. The surgeon will state the amount of weight that is to be applied in both instances (the patient may be weighed before the application of traction so that the doctor can, more accurately, assess the amount of weight required). For specific care of patients on traction see Chapter 2. Union of the femoral shaft takes approximately three months.

■ Cast brace

A cast brace is frequently used in treating a mid-shaft or distal fracture of the femur. A cast brace has three components:

1 A snug plaster is applied to increase the hydrodynamic compressive effect of the thigh muscle and to provide for immobilization of the fractured fragments.

   The plaster is referred to as a 'thigh cuff' and extends as far up the thigh as possible and down to the knee joint.

2 Two hinges are inserted into the plaster to allow active motion of the knee joint. The hinges also connect the thigh cuff to the short leg cast.

3 A walking cast or a cylinder cast is applied below the knee to provide support for the thigh cuff and it prevents the thigh cuff from slipping distally.

The cast brace is applied after swelling has reduced and when the soft tissues have started to heal. Proper alignment must have been established first – this can take between two to six weeks following injury. The patient will have been in skeletal traction prior to the application of a cast brace. Suitable analgesia should be given prior to the application. The advantage of having a cast brace is that it permits the patient to weight-bear early. Patients also maintain a fairly normal gait because the hip joint and the knee joint are free to move. Patients are able to get in and out of bed and chairs without too much difficulty.

It is advisable to show patients a photograph of a cast brace before it is applied as they are often very anxious about what the cast will look like.

Information should be given regarding the type of shoes the patient should wear. Occasionally a shoe worn on the uninvolved leg has to be built up to match the length of the involved leg.

■ Fractured femur in babies and infants

Fractured shaft of femur sometimes occurs as a result of a difficult delivery. In infants under the age of three years treatment is by means of gallows traction (Bryant's traction). This is achieved by applying skin extensions to the infant's legs (both legs). The extension tapes are then tied securely to a frame fixed over the cot. The baby lies on his back and hangs by his legs as it were to an overhead beam, with his buttocks just clearing the cot (Fig. 6).

The maintenance and management of the traction applies as stated in Chapter 2. Circulation, mobility and sensation to the feet must be closely observed and any abnormalities reported immediately to the surgeon. Sciatic nerve damage is a possible, but rare, complication.

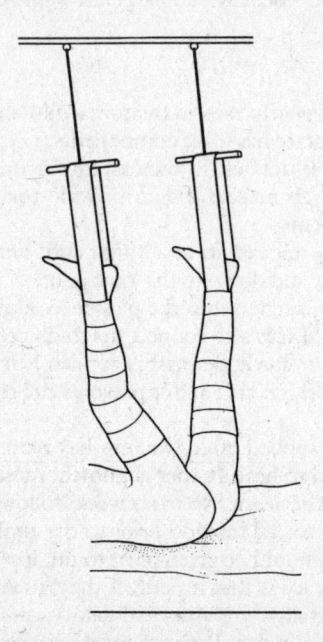

Fig. 6 Gallows (Bryant's) traction

Nursing management of the infant should be appropriate to the age, with sufficient stimulation in the environment. Care is needed with feeding the baby in this position and the mother may be initially apprehensive about this. Nappies can be placed beneath the buttocks and care of the baby's skin in this region can be continued by washing the skin followed by application of a barrier cream, such as petroleum jelly (soft paraffin) or zinc and castor oil. The baby will obviously have to be washed in bed and the mother may like to do this. It is often necessary for the baby to remain on gallows traction for up to four weeks.

■ Fractured tibia and fibula

Fractures of the tibia and fibula are often compound. Motor cycle accidents often result in the above fractures accompanied by damage to the soft tissues. (See management of compound fracture page 35.) Reduction may be achieved by manipulation and the application of a plaster of Paris cast. Skeletal traction may be effected by the insertion of a pin through the lower end of the tibial shaft and the limb then encased in a plaster cast extending from the toes to the groin. This in turn is supported on a form of splintage, e.g. flexed Thomas' bed splint or a Braun splint (Fig. 7).

■ Pott's fracture

This is a fracture-dislocation of the ankle joint with damage to the ligaments. Either one or both malleoli may be fractured with displacement of the talus. Treatment is reduction and immobilization in the position appropriate to the injury. The patient may be allowed to walk in the plaster, weight-bearing in four to six weeks depending on the severity of

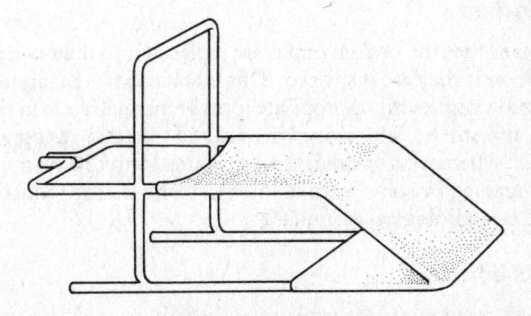

Fig. 7 Braun splint

the fracture. Some fractures may require open reduction and internal fixation.

■ Fractured pelvis

Stable fractures of the pelvis are not usually serious and are generally treated by bed rest for a few days. If the fractures are unstable they can be serious because of the possible complications. Internal haemorrhage is a possibility, as well as damage to the organs within the pelvis, e.g. bladder, urethra, vagina, uterus. Close observation of the vital signs: pulse and blood pressure in particular, urinary output, the amount and colour, are noted and recorded. Treatment for any internal injuries is given priority over the fracture, and the girth may be measured at regular intervals.

Depending on the type of fracture the patient may be nursed in a pelvic suspensory sling. In some cases manipulation may be required and immobilization in a double hip plaster spica. Leg traction may have to be applied. Analgesia is required for pain and bed rest is usually continued for 8 to 12 weeks.

■ PRINCIPLES OF TREATMENT AND MANAGEMENT OF PATIENTS WITH FRACTURES

The principles of treatment include:
a reducing the fracture
b maintaining immobilization
c restoration of function.

■ Reduction

This means that the broken bones are replaced into their correct anatomical position if they are displaced. This is achieved by manipulation, when the surgeon applies the appropriate form of manual traction under general or local anaesthetic. This is known as closed reduction as opposed to open reduction when operative means are required for reducing the fracture and is accompanied by some form of internal fixation. The reduction is always checked by radiological examination.

■ Immobilization

Once reduction has been achieved and the bone ends are in good alignment, some form of immobilization is required to maintain this position.

Fractures reduced by the closed method are immobilized by external splintage, such as plaster of Paris, splints, traction. Some form of external splintage is sometimes required following internal fixation such as plates, screws, bone grafts, intramedullary nails.

A further radiological examination will be carried out to make certain that the reduction is still in good alignment.

■ Restoration of function

While immobilization of the fracture is necessary, exercise and movement of those parts not immobilized are important. It is usual therefore to encourage the active use of all those joints not immobilized, and the physiotherapist will teach the patient suitable exercises designed to maintain muscle strength.

■ Pain

Fractures are always accompanied by pain, and suitable analgesia should be prescribed.

■ Compound fractures

Fractures accompanied by wounds increase the risk of infection. It is usual for the patient to receive an injection of tetanus vaccine and possibly Humotet (human tetanus immunoglobulin). A course of antibiotics is also prescribed and administered. The wound will require toileting and possibly excision of damaged tissue. Reduction of the fracture will take place at the same time together with the appropriate form of immobilization.

Compound fractures may or may not be treated by open reduction and internal fixation. Whichever method is adopted to treat the fracture the management of the wound is undertaken as a matter of urgency.

■ Shock

Patients admitted to hospital with fractures may be in a state of shock and may be haemorrhaging, either internally or externally. Frequent and close observations of the vital signs, urinary output and general appearance of the patient must be made. A specimen of blood will be obtained for grouping and cross-matching and intravenous therapy commenced. The relevant radiological examination(s) will be carried out.

■ Emergency admission

Patients with fractures are admitted as emergencies, therefore a record of valuables and property will have to be made, according to the hospital policy, and steps taken to contact the patient's next of kin, unless they are accompanying the patient.

■ Recovery

Following the initial treatment the patient, depending on the type of fracture and extent of injuries, may have to spend some time in hospital. When reduction and immobilization are achieved patients usually feel quite well in themselves within a few days. It is then a matter of keeping them appropriately occupied and preventing complications such as chest infection, deep venous thrombosis, depression, urinary tract infections and renal calculi.

Specific complications of fractures include: non-union; mal-union; fat embolism; injuries to nerves, blood vessels and organs; joint stiffness, adhesions and myositis ossificans. (Care of splintage is discussed in Chapter 2.)

Depending on the type of fracture and severity the surgeon will decide when the patient can be allowed up either non-weight-bearing or bearing weight. A low-heel walking shoe is worn on the unaffected limb. A walking plaster requires reinforcement. The patient may then be allowed home when he is mobile on crutches or sticks. He should be given clear directions as to what he may or may not do; he should also be told when to return for follow-up and what to do if any difficulties arise.

■ PRACTICE QUESTIONS

1 *What is meant by the following terms?*
  a Osteocyte
  b Periosteum
  c The Haversian system
  d Callus formation
  e Compound fracture
  f Complicated fracture
  g Impacted fracture
  h The reduction of a fracture
  i Volkmann's ischaemic contracture
  j Myositis ossificans
  k Colles' fracture
  l Intertrochanteric fracture of femur
  m Flexion contracture of a joint
  n Intramedullary nail
  o Non-union

p Slow union
q Mal-union
r Crepitus
s Fat embolism
t Open reduction and internal fixation.

2 *Briefly explain the following:*
  a Why is wound toilet and excision necessary following a compound fracture?
  b Why is a form of immobilization necessary following a fracture? State the possible ways in which this can be achieved.
  c Describe the signs and symptoms which may arise as a result of a fat embolism.
  d What factors may lead to joint stiffness and adhesions following the treatment of fractures?
  e Describe the sequence of events that take place in the process of bone healing.
  f Explain how activity is maintained during the period of immobilization leading to eventual restoration of function.
  g Following injury to the region of the elbow, i.e. lower end of humerus, and upper end of the forearm, the patient may have to remain in hospital until it is certain that circulation to the limb is adequate. Why is this so?
  h Why are intracapsular fractures of the femoral neck often treated by replacing the head of the femur with a prosthesis?
  i Describe what measures you would take to prevent the development of pressure sores in an elderly person following a fractured neck of femur.
  j What exercises would be encouraged for a patient following plaster of Paris immobilization for Colles' fracture?

3 *Answer the following questions True or False:*
  a The osteoblasts are found in the innermost layer of periosteum.
  b A fracture which damages nerves, blood vessels, and penetrates organs is called a comminuted fracture.
  c A greenstick fracture is commonly seen in children.
  d Eight small bones make up the carpus (wrist bones).
  e The scapula is commonly known as the collar bone.
  f The lateral malleolus is the lower end of the tibia.
  g Posture, hormones, genetic factors and dietary factors affect bone growth and development.
  h The red bone marrow is found in compact bone.
  i Diaphysis is the term used for the shaft of a long bone.
  j The epiphysis is the part of bone in which growth takes place.

Answers

1 *a* A bone cell.
   b A fibrous outer covering of bone.
   c A series of small interconnecting channels found in compact bone supplying the bone cells with oxygen and nutrients.
   d Tissue which develops at the fracture site eventually forming new bone. Callus formation can be observed on radiographs.
   e A fracture accompanied by a wound when there is contact between the fracture and the external environment.
   f A fracture which involves damage to other structures such as nerves and viscera.
   g Where one fragment of the fracture is driven into the other.
   h Restoring the correct anatomical alignment of the bone so that it may heal in the correct position.
   i Lack of blood supply to the muscles of the forearm and hand causing contracture deformities when the brachial artery is damaged or compressed following injury.
   j Post-traumatic ossification of a haematoma around a joint. Cause is unknown. The most usual site is at the elbow joint. Treatment is rest.
   k Fracture of the lower end of the radius.
   l A fracture in the trochanteric region of the femur. Such fractures are extracapsular and do not interfere with the supply of blood to the femoral head.
   m When the flexor muscles retain a joint in a particular position.
   n A nail which is inserted along the length of the medullary cavity as a means of immobilizing a fracture, e.g. Küntscher nail for fractured shaft of femur.
   o Following reduction and a period of immobilization a fracture fails to unite.
   p When a fracture takes longer than is usual or expected for that particular type of fracture to heal.
   q When a fracture unites but the position in which it has healed is incorrect. This may or may not interfere with the function of the part.
   r A 'grating' sensation which may be felt or heard when two rough edges rub together.
   s A complication of a fracture which may be due to the release of fat from the bone marrow cavity.
   t When a fracture is reduced surgically and some form of internal splintage (plates, screws, nails) is used to maintain the reduction.

2 *a* To prevent/reduce the development of infection as dead tissue is an ideal medium for the multiplication of organisms.

b A period of immobilization is usually necessary to maintain the reduction so allowing the fracture to heal. This can be achieved by
  - external splintage, plaster cast, splints, traction.
  - internal splintage, i.e. fixing the reduction by means of metal plates, screws and so on, at the time of surgery.

  A form of external splintage may also be used as well as internal fixation.

c As with any other embolism it depends on where the embolism lodges. The patient may be pyrexial, have tachycardia and some difficulty in breathing – a dotted fine rash may appear on the shoulders and pectoral regions.

d When damaged joints are moved too early before tissues have had time to heal. Passively stretching a stiff joint. Inadequate exercise to those joints not immobilized. Inadequate exercise of joints when immobilization has been discontinued.

e Bleeding at the fracture site – clot formation. Invasion of the clot by new blood capillaries and bone-forming cells – callus formation – development of new bone – reshaping.

f Movement of those joints not immobilized in the splintage.

  Isometric (static) exercises may be ordered for those parts affected.

  As soon as possible the patient is taught to use the limb that is immobilized, i.e. while still in plaster. For example, a walking plaster will be provided for the patient with a lower limb fracture.

  Active exercises of the affected limb are performed when the period of immobilization is over.

g Damage to the brachial artery may cause Volkmann's ischaemic contracture. The radial pulse is palpated frequently and any pain, swelling, change in colour or temperature of the hand is reported to the surgeon without any delay.

h Because the blood supply to the femoral head may be interrupted causing necrosis of the head and non-union of the fracture.

i Regular change of the patient's position, or, alternatively, frequent relief of pressure by lifting the patient slightly off the mattress.

  Sufficient number of nurses to lift the patient so that he is not dragged along the bed, and a nurse available to maintain the position of the limb. This also applies to the placing and removing of bedpans, changing sheets, draw sheets and so on.

  Appropriate selection of aids, to help prevent the development of sores e.g. sheepskin. 'Monkey pole' provided so that patient can help with lifts.

  Frequent checks made of the skin particularly those areas subjected to pressure.

Keeping the skin clean and dry and the bed linen beneath the patient should be kept smooth and crease free.

Ensure that the patient takes an adequate nourishing diet and ample fluid intake.

j The plaster cast for a Colles' fracture extends from the knuckles to just below the elbow. The shoulder and elbow joints are exercised and the patient is encouraged to exercise the fingers, i.e. touching the palm with the tips of the fingers and fully extending the fingers and spreading them out. The patient is also told to touch the tip of each finger in turn with the tip of the thumb. The patient should also be shown how to abduct and internally and externally rotate the shoulder joint, i.e. placing the arm behind the back and behind the neck respectively.

3 *a* True
  b False
  c True
  d True
  e False
  f False
  g True
  h False
  i True
  j True.

4 Spine and spinal injuries

The objectives of this section are to:
1 Outline the structure of the spine.
2 List common conditions affecting the spine.
3 Describe the management of patients who have sustained injury to the spinal cord.

The spinal column is made up of 33 individual bones called the vertebrae, and is divided into five regions namely:
1 *Cervical* – 7 vertebrae – secondary curve.
   The first two vertebrae of the cervical region are called the atlas and the axis and are designed to allow movement of the skull on the vertebral column, e.g. nodding.
2 *Thoracic* (dorsal) – 12 vertebrae – primary curve.
   The 12 pairs of ribs articulate with each thoracic vertebra. Exaggeration of this curve is called kyphosis.
3 *Lumbar* – 5 vertebrae – secondary curve.
   The vertebra in this region are large and are designed to bear the weight of the trunk. Exaggeration of this curve is called lordosis.
4 *Sacral* (sacrum) – 5 vertebrae – primary curve.
   The sacral vertebrae are fused to form one bone (the sacrum).
5 *Coccygeal* (coccyx) – 4 vertebrae which are fused.

Each vertebra consists of a body anteriorly which articulates with the body of the vertebra above and below by means of a cartilaginous joint; a spinous process posteriorly (this is the bony protuberance which can be palpated) and two transverse processes (Fig. 8). In between the vertebral bodies are intervertebral discs. The outer covering of the disc is termed the annulus fibrosus (fibrocartilage) in which is contained the nucleus pulposus. The discs are connected to the vertebral bodies by means of hyaline cartilage.

Muscles are attached to the transverse processes and spinal process.

The vertebral column forms the vertebral canal through which runs the spinal cord. It extends from the foramen magnum to the upper borders of the second lumbar vertebra. The spinal nerves leave the spinal cord through the intervertebral foramina.

The movements possible in the spinal column include flexion, extension, lateral flexion and rotation.

42 *Orthopaedic Nursing*

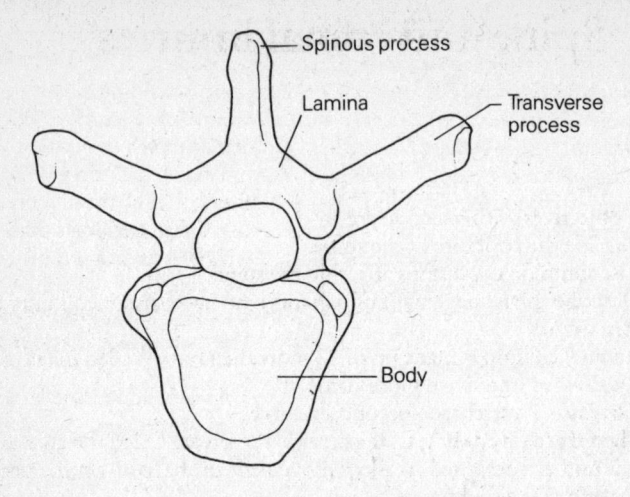

Fig. 8 A vertebra

The upright posture is maintained by the extensor muscles of the back.

□ *Low back pain*
This is a common complaint and while it may be due to one of several causes, such as trauma to the soft tissue structures, straining of ligaments and muscles and spraining the lumbar-sacral joint, postural defects, congenital abnormalities affecting the vertebral column, malignant disease and gynaecological conditions in females; the most common cause is a prolapsed intervertebral disc.

■ PROLAPSED INTERVERTEBRAL DISC IN THE LUMBAR REGION

Low back pain is produced by the nucleus pulposus protruding through the ruptured annulus fibrosus. Depending on the extent of the protrusion the nerve roots in the region may be compressed, giving rise to sciatica: that is pain referred along the sciatic nerve. The patient will complain of pain down the back of the leg to the ankle and outer aspect of the foot to the little toe. The pain may be accompanied by numbness and tingling of the foot or calf on the affected side. The ankle jerk may be absent, the patient has difficulty in flexing the lumbar spine forward and straight leg raising is painful and limited. On examination the doctor may observe a scoliosis and flattening of the normal lumbar lordosis.

The patient may give a history of low back pain extending over a number of years with more recent onset of sciatica. Some however experience the immediate onset of sciatica following a sudden acute strain on the back.

Investigations include radiological examination, including CT scan, myelogram; blood examination; and, sometimes, a lumbar puncture.

Conservative treatment may consist of rest on a firm bed for a period of, perhaps, up to six weeks; pelvic or leg traction; a plaster jacket followed by the wearing of a Goldthwaite belt or a surgical corset.

Manipulations following the principles of different schools of practice (Cyriax, Maitland) can be highly effective. They are usually carried out by experienced physiotherapists.

Patients who do not respond to conservative treatment may require surgery when removal of the ruptured disc is carried out by means of laminectomy.

■ Management of the patient undergoing laminectomy

The preparation of the patient is similar to that prior to any major surgical procedure. Consent is obtained from the patient, blood is grouped and cross-matched; radiological examination and other relevant investigations will already have been carried out. The back will require shaving from the shoulders to the buttocks. If a bone graft is to be taken the donor site may have to be prepared also. The physiotherapist will teach the patient breathing exercises and spinal exercises for continuing after surgery. A baseline is noted of the vital signs and the doctor will carry out a medical and neurological examination before surgery. He will also explain the procedure to the patient and give him some idea of what to expect following the surgery; the nurse should be prepared to reinforce this information and answer any further questions that the patient might have. The anaesthetist will visit the patient also.

The night prior to surgery the bowels are evacuated, if necessary by an enema or suppositories. Nothing is given orally for six hours before surgery. Sedation may be prescribed to ensure a good night's rest.

□ *Postoperative management*

The patient is nursed in a bed with a firm base; the maintenance of a clear airway and the observation of vital signs are maintained.

Positioning of the patient is important and will be as requested by the surgeon. The alignment of the spine must be maintained and the patient turned in one piece from side to supine to side ('log rolling', see below). When he is able to turn himself he must also maintain the alignment of the spine and prevent any strain on the back muscles. The patient's skin and pressure areas are observed frequently as well as sensation and mobility of the lower limbs. The wound dressing is observed for bleeding or cerebrospinal fluid leakage. Analgesia is administered as prescribed.

Attention is paid to the urinary output as urinary retention may be a problem. It is sometimes necessary to catheterize a patient. If a catheter is not inserted the female patient may use a female urinal or receiver to avoid lifting on to a bedpan.

Depending on the surgeon some patients may be allowed up on the second or third day. Care is taken to maintain the alignment of the spine on getting out of bed and a support may sometimes be ordered. The patient is helped and supervised getting out of bed initially and the length of time spent out sitting and walking is gradually increased as the patient improves. If a fusion operation has been performed the patient may have to remain in bed for a longer period.

Prior to discharge the patient is advised regarding postural exercises and is taught to lift safely. Swimming may be resumed.

The patient is followed up by the surgeon and will be advised about returning to work.

■ Log rolling

Patients with spinal injuries and back problems can be moved easily by this procedure:
1 Remove all the patient's pillows.
2 Ask the patient to cross his arms across his chest.
3 If possible three nurses should move the patient but it is acceptable for two nurses to log roll a patient. The nurses stand on the same side of the patient's bed. The nurses place their hands under the patient's shoulders, back, buttocks and legs for support and carefully lift the patient to one side of the bed.
4 One nurse goes to the other side of the bed. A covered pillow is placed between the patient's legs.
5 The patient keeps his arms crossed and one nurse helps the patient to roll by supporting his buttocks and back as he turns away from her.
6 The other nurse/nurses on the other side of the bed provide additional support for the patient where necessary.
7 The patient's position is maintained and the nurse at the back of the patient repositions the pillows for support. The pillow under the patient's head is replaced. One pillow remains between the patient's knees while he is on his side. Two pillows support the patient's back and buttocks. Finally one pillow can be placed in front of the patient's chest to support his arm.

■ INJURIES TO THE SPINE

Injuries to the spine consist of fractures which may or may not damage the spinal cord. Unstable fractures of the spine may lead to spinal cord injury and render the patient paralysed. All injuries to the spine are considered unstable until otherwise determined. Fractures of the vertebra without involvement of the spinal cord are treated according to the type of fracture and its location. Fractures in any part of the spine may require open reduction and internal fixation. Otherwise conservative methods are adopted including skull traction for a fracture-dislocation of the cervical spine. Bed rest may be all that is required for fractures in the lumbar region. Some fractures may require immobilization in a plaster jacket.

■ Spinal cord injury

If a patient is suspected of having sustained injury to the spine it is important that he is handled very carefully and is lifted and turned in 'one piece', that is, the spine is not flexed or rotated in any way, as damage to the cord can occur as a result of incorrectly handling the patient. If possible the patient should be treated in a spinal injury unit.

The extent of the paralysis depends on the level of the lesion; that is, the loss of function will be of the parts of the body supplied by the spinal nerves below the level of the lesion. The spinal cord serves as a pathway for sensory and motor nerves, as well as the autonomic nervous system; thus there can be loss of movement and sensation. Bowel and bladder control and sexual function (particularly in men) may all be affected as is vasomotor control.

Paralysis from the waist down is termed paraplegia. Paralysis from the neck down, that is all four limbs and the trunk is termed tetraplegia or quadriplegia. Injuries of the cervical spine result in tetraplegia. Injuries may be sustained at work, e.g. falling from a height, or a heavy load falling on to the person, road traffic accidents, and sporting activities, e.g. diving into shallow water, Rugby football, trampolining and so on.

The initial treatment of the patient depends on his condition and the level of the lesion. The patient may have multiple injuries; the lesion may be high cervical, resulting in respiratory difficulties necessitating a tracheostomy and assisted ventilation.

The aim of all treatment involves the management of the fracture, prevention of complications and rehabilitation leading ultimately to independence. Total independence *can* be achieved by the paraplegic patient, but the degree of independence achieved by the tetraplegic is dependent on the level of the lesion. The higher the lesion the more dependent the patient is likely to be.

Fractures

Alignment and stability to the spinal column is achieved by reducing the fracture. This may be done by postural reduction – positioning patients correctly by means of pillows, hyperextending the appropriate part of the spine. Occasionally the positions required for reduction are flexion or neutral depending on the position of the fracture. Skull traction may be used for fracture-dislocation of the cervical spine. Open reduction and internal fixation may also be employed.

NURSING MANAGEMENT

The patient who has sustained injury to the spinal cord is vulnerable to complications and nursing management is of the utmost importance. Teamwork is a must with the surgeon in charge of the spinal unit, possibly a urologist, the nursing staff, medical social worker, physiotherapists, occupational therapists, radiographers all involved.

The most important member of this team is the patient himself who should be involved with his own management. The patient has to develop an awareness of the importance of aspects of his care because eventually he will care for himself; this includes the importance of positioning, of changing position, of drinking at least 3 litres a day and so on. This awareness is developed as part of the rehabilitation programme, and each patient knows the level of his lesion.

It has already been stated that spinal injury units exist to manage patients who have sustained spinal cord injury. The advantage of such units is that those caring for the patient recognize the special needs of the paraplegic and tetraplegic. Patients in the unit will include new patients who have recently acquired spinal injuries, those in the various stages of rehabilitation and those who have returned for reassessment or treatment of a complication.

The number of beds on a spinal injury ward tends to be fewer than the average acute general ward, because the dependency level of some of the patients at any given time is quite high. The number of nursing staff should be adequate for turning patients and this is one procedure that is *never* neglected on a spinal unit. On the hour and every hour, *day* and *night* a patient will require turning and nothing must interfere with this. This strict routine, however, does not detract from the individuality of the patient. Both nursing staff and patients are aware of the need to relieve pressure to avoid the development of sores.

From the early days on the spinal unit the patient meets people from various disciplines who will participate in his rehabilitation programme. Relatives can become involved in the management of the patient; are kept informed of the patient's condition; and may be taught certain aspects of the patient's care at the appropriate time. It must be recognized that relatives require support and time to talk through their feelings and understanding of the situation. The prospect, for instance, of caring for a husband who had become a tetraplegic creates a situation which is charged with fear and mixed feelings, for many different reasons. The process of coping, trying to understand, trying to reason, for both the patient and the relative is a gradual, continuing process that extends through the rehabilitation period and beyond. The nurses on the spinal unit recognize that both the patient and his relatives vary in the way they cope with their situation.

■ Positioning of the patient

Positioning of the patient in bed is of the utmost importance, both in relation to the reduction of the fracture and the prevention of complications, such as pressure sore formation, joint contractures and drop foot. Many pillows are used for this purpose. They are carefully placed and positioned, and the patient is nursed naked. Cradles may be used to relieve the weight of the bed clothes. A body sheet may be placed next to the patient to ensure that he is kept warm. Pillows are arranged directly on the

Bony prominences are protected from pressure

Feet are maintained at right angles to the legs

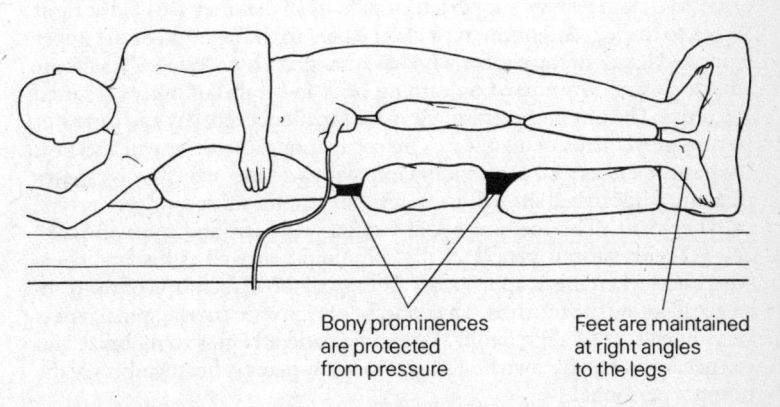

Fig. 9 Positioning the paralysed patient by using pillows

mattress beneath the patient so that the bony prominences are not subjected to any pressure. Pillows are placed at the foot end of the bed supported against a board to maintain the feet in a correct position to prevent the development of drop foot (Fig. 9). When the patient is turned, the pillows are removed, turned over, and the covers changed as and when required.

Hyperextension of the spine can be achieved by the use of double pillows or in the case of a cervical spine a small roll placed beneath the neck. The bed itself must have a firm base; if such beds are not available, fracture boards will be required. Electric beds are available and greatly facilitate the turning of a patient but it must be stressed that the use of such a bed does not replace the need to observe the patient's skin and bony prominences frequently.

The patient usually remains on bed rest for a period of up to approximately 12 weeks. This leaves much time for thinking and returning to that split second when the course of his whole life was changed. It is not unusual to find when interrupting a patient deep in thought that he makes reference to the time of injury.

Initially, following injury, the patient is turned every hour or perhaps two, later this can be extended to three hours. Nothing is allowed to prevent these turns being carried out. Several nurses are required to turn the patient, and the nurse leading the team will initiate each lift in turn. If skull traction is present another nurse, usually the team leader, supports the head during the turns. The patient must be moved in one piece and the alignment of the spine maintained throughout. When the patient is on his side his lower leg is flexed at the hip and the knee, the upper leg is held in extension, both feet are supported by pillows so that they are held at right angles to the leg. Attention must also be paid to the position of the upper limbs and hands of the patient who has sustained a high lesion. Patients are almost always now nursed on turning beds and teams of nurses are used less often. The physiotherapist will visit the patient every day and carry out passive movements of all joints. The occupational therapist will also visit the patient and as well as providing him with activities which he is capable of doing while in bed she will assess him later for the most appropriate type of wheelchair. The medical social worker will visit and she will make contact with various people in the community as well as his employers where and when this is appropriate. It is usual for all members of the team to get to know the relatives. The concept of teamwork in the spinal unit is very much that of a big family. When the patient begins to mobilize and can get around on his own he also gets to know many other members of the hospital personnel.

■ Eating and drinking

The patient will be given a well-balanced nutritious diet and plenty of fluids. The paraplegic patient, although in the supine position, after some practice will be able to feed himself. Flexible straws for drinking are very useful. The tetraplegic patient will require feeding and help with drinking while he is in bed. Later when in a wheelchair every effort will be made for the patient to feed himself sitting at the table. The occupational therapist will assess the patient's need for aids to help him become independent. Relatives are encouraged to help with feeding at an early stage and often arrange to come at mealtimes so that they can involve themselves. The patient is made aware from the early stage that drinking enough is important. Water jugs on the lockers are refilled several times during the course of the day and it does not take very long before the patient points out that his water jug is empty! Again when mobilized in a wheelchair the patient will refill his own jug.

■ Breathing

The maintenance of a good general nutritious state of the patient and frequent turns will help to prevent the complication of a chest infection. Tetraplegic patients require special mention, because a high lesion affects respiratory muscles and, therefore, the patient's ability to cough. Sometimes a tracheostomy is required as well as assisted breathing. Chest physiotherapy is of the utmost importance as the patient is susceptible to the development of chest complications. Antibiotic therapy is usually prescribed by the doctor, should the patient develop any signs of an upper respiratory tract infection.

■ Hygiene and care of the skin

While the patient is on bed rest he is washed by the nurses. The paraplegic can wash his own face and hands and after a few days can shave himself. Special attention is paid to the state of the skin and the patient is handled gently at all times. The genital region is washed and dried. The tetraplegic patient will require total care by the nurses but depending on the amount of movement he has in his upper limbs he eventually may also manage to wash his face. Once in a wheelchair the paraplegic patient will be able to care for his own personal hygiene.

Patients who are managed on spinal units do not usually develop pressure sores because the principle of relieving pressure at frequent intervals over the 24-hour period is closely adhered to all times. However, patients may be admitted to the unit for the treatment of sores. This is based on the principle of prevention, that is relief of pressure. The patient is nursed in bed and kept off the sore/sores. If several sores are present it may be necessary to use large sorbo packs placed in such a way that all bony prominences are relieved of pressure as well as the sores, whether the patient is in the lateral position, or supine. The prone position may also be used. The pressure sore is treated by excision of any necrotic tissue and slough, and a dressing applied. Appropriate solutions are used to clean the sores and some may require packing. It is generally considered that what is actually used on a pressure sore for its treatment is immaterial, as long as the patient's weight is kept off it. When the sore is healed the patient is allowed up again and the importance of preventing more sores is further reinforced. At the same time as treating the sore the general condition of the patient is not overlooked and anaemia may be treated by a blood transfusion. Diet high in protein is given and vitamin supplements may also be prescribed. Occasionally sores may require plastic surgery.

In the acute stage of injury while the patient is nursed in bed the nails are kept clean and short. The hair is kept clean and washed in bed. The paraplegic patient can clean his own teeth but requires a nurse to hold the receptacle for swilling the mouth. The nurse will have to clean the teeth of a patient who is tetraplegic.

■ Elimination

□ *Management of the bladder*

Management of the bladder varies from unit to unit and from patient to patient. In some instances a method of intermittent catheterization is adopted after the first 12–24 hours following injury. In other instances a method of continuous catheterization is adopted using a self-retaining catheter. Whichever method is adopted the aim is to prevent the development of urinary tract infection, hydronephrosis and renal damage. An intravenous urogram (pyelogram) (IVU, IVP) is not considered urgent but is usually carried out at some stage during the period of hospitalization. It is hoped that eventually the patient will be continent without the continued use of a catheter. Scrupulous cleanliness is required in the management of the catheter and a strict aseptic technique employed during its insertion. If an automatic bladder is present it may be possible to train this so that emptying occurs as a result of some external stimulus. Alternatively, the bladder may be devoid of muscle activity (autonomous) and may be emptied by manual expression, that is exerting manual pressure over the lower part of the abdomen. Management of the bladder and achievement of some control requires much patience on the part of those caring for the patient as well as the patient himself. Measurement of the residual urine has to be done at frequent intervals during the course of bladder training. Sometimes the urethral sphincter does not relax properly with a resulting high residual urine and stagnation in the bladder. This may have to be treated by a sphincterotomy which will render the patient incontinent. The male patient manages subsequently by wearing a condom which is attached to a drainage bag while in bed, and attached by tubing to a bag worn on the inside of the lower part of the leg underneath trousers when in a chair. This prevents back pressure of urine on the kidneys and stagnation of urine in the bladder. Some patients may continue with the use of catheters. Female patients are sometimes managed by transplanting the ureters into a portion of the ileum and bringing this on to the abdominal wall (ileal conduit) and a bag is then worn under the clothes. Eventually the paraplegic patient will be able to manage his own bladder, care of condoms, bags and so on; the tetraplegic patient will require some assistance.

□ *Bowels*
Bedpans are never used. The aim of bowel management is to bring about the evacuation of formed stools, regularly. This is usually done at the same time of the day, i.e. mornings/evenings daily or alternate days by the use of suppositories. Following the insertion of two glycerine suppositories, a large incontinent or gamgee pad is placed beneath the patient and the bowel content is expelled on to the pad. The pad is then removed and the patient cleaned. If an anal reflex is not present suppositories cannot be retained in the rectum, and the patient's bowels are evacuated manually. Eventually the paraplegic patient will be able to manage his own bowels, insert suppositories and transfer himself on to the toilet using an inflatable rubber toilet seat. Tetraplegic patients will require assistance. Relatives may be taught to help patients with bowel management, but sometimes the patient prefers the relative (perhaps a husband or wife) not to perform the procedure, in which case alternative arrangements are made with the community nurses.

■ **Mobilization**

The surgeon will decide when the patient is allowed up depending on the radiographs and the patient's condition. Once it is decided, he is gradually sat up in bed before getting out into a chair. When the patient gets up continued support may be required for the fracture, e.g. a collar may have to be worn for a few weeks. The tetraplegic patient may experience fainting when he gets in a chair because of the vasomotor disturbance; when this happens it is necessary to tilt the chair back and raise the patient's legs. An abdominal binder may be applied if the postural hypotension continues to be a problem.

Because there is still the possibility of pressure sore formation patients are taught to lift themselves off the chair at regular intervals. Tetraplegic patients will require lifting regularly by the nurses. A cushion (e.g. ripple, sorbo rubber) is usually placed in the wheelchair. Physiotherapy is continued in the department and the patient learns to balance and transfer and carry out strengthening exercises as well as standing.

Following rehabilitation the *paraplegic* patient should be totally independent. He will be able to dress himself, transfer from bed to chair, chair to bath, chair to toilet and so on. He will check his own skin by the use of mirrors, turn himself in bed and arrange his own pillows. He will participate in sporting activities, swimming, table tennis, archery and so on. He will attend the occupational therapy department, and the possibilities of returning to work, or alternative work and retraining will be discussed with the patient.

The *tetraplegic* patient will be mobilized and rehabilitated in the same way but the degree of independence achieved is dependent largely on how high the lesion is and how much strength the patient has in his upper limbs. Some tetraplegic patients will be able to manoeuvre a wheelchair quite effectively if they have reasonable strength in their arms, with grip pads applied to the palms of the hands. Others will not be able to manoeuvre a wheelchair with their arms and will require an electrically-powered wheelchair operated by an appropriate type of possum device. Some will be able to dress and get in and out of bed with assistance. Others will require lifting by the nurses from bed to chair and so on. During this active period of rehabilitation the relatives are positively involved in the management, with a view to helping the patient when he gets home. Adaptations may be required in the home, e.g. ramps, stair lifts, rails, doorways widened and so on. The tetraplegic patient will always require some degree of assistance, and will have to continue to be turned in bed after going home.

■ **Psychological considerations**

It is understandable that during the course of hospitalization and rehabilitation there will be times when the patient feels depressed about the whole situation. It is a process that the patient must be allowed to work through and cope with in whatever way is best for him. Staff and patients on spinal units tend to get to know each other very well so that things like discussing difficulties or wanting to be left alone to think things through can often be anticipated. Outbursts are sometimes encountered and each and every patient manifests his frustrations in different ways.

The patient in a wheelchair is at a distinct disadvantage in having to look up at everybody when speaking to them. It is useful for nursing staff to sit/kneel to the patient's level rather than stand over the patient when discussing something with him. Understandably the patient does not take kindly to being patronized and this should always be avoided. Some people make the error of assuming that physically disabled persons are mentally disabled.

It is difficult for nurses to stand back and watch a patient struggling to dress or to manoeuvre a wheelchair up an incline, but to intervene all the time is ultimately to do the patient a disservice. If he is to achieve independence he must be allowed to do as much as he can himself – and this frequently involves much effort.

While in the spinal unit the patient is safe and secure in the sense that he is with other patients who are like himself and those caring for him are familiar with the difficulties he encounters. However, preparations have to be made for the patient to move out of this small circle, to be with his family and the community from which he came. Like everything else this is done gradually, and the appropriate timing of these events is very important. The first encounter outside the unit may be an evening out with family, friends or/and perhaps a member of staff. Whoever accompanies the patient will have to remember that this can be a very frightening experience for him; for the first time the outside world – parts of it which were previously familiar to the patient – will be viewed from a wheelchair. The patient may then spend a day at home accompanied by a member of staff and those persons whose help will be required from the community may also be contacted so that they can visit the home at the same time. The patient may then spend a weekend at home, so that he and the family are gradually introduced to what will be expected of them and any problems which may arise can be ironed out before he is finally discharged home. Patients require much information about obtaining different kinds of appliances and equipment, which departments are responsible for what, and it may take some time for the patient to familiarize himself with all this. The patient and his relatives are made very aware that they can contact the spinal unit at any time no matter how trivial they may feel the difficulties are.

Different problems will be encountered at different times throughout their lives as they do with able-bodied people, but the paraplegic/tetraplegic patient needs to be aware that organizations do exist, and whereas they may not be directly able to help with a particular problem, they can direct the patient to those who can. Couples can be offered counselling regarding sex, adoption and artificial insemination. The general practitioner is informed of the patient's discharge home – indeed he should have been involved from the earliest possible time for he can arrange many of the community services which will be required, for example district nurse, health visitor, provision of appliances, and so on.

Paraplegics and tetraplegics and their families may like to know about the Spinal Injuries Association whose address is 5 Crowndale Road, London NW1 1TU.

■ PRACTICE QUESTIONS

1 *What is meant by the following terms?*
   a Laminectomy
   b Prolapsed intervertebral disc
   c Paraplegia
   d Tetraplegia
   e Autonomous bladder
   f Possum device
   g Slough
   h Sphincterotomy
   i Residual urine
   j Anal reflex.
2 *Explain briefly the following:*
   a Why after approximately six weeks may the patient be turned 3-hourly instead of 2-hourly?
   b What is meant by postural reduction of the fractured spine?
   c Why is it important to prevent the development of complications in a patient who has damage to the spinal cord?
   d What are spasms and contractures?
3 *Mark the following True or False*
   a A person becomes paraplegic following a spinal fracture.
   b An injury below the level of T12 would cause paralysis (partial/complete) of the legs, bowel and bladder.
   c There are seven cervical vertebrae and therefore seven cervical nerves.
   d The diaphragm is supplied by the phrenic nerve which leaves the spinal cord at the level of C4.
   e The spinal cord extends from the foramen magnum to the level of the 3rd lumbar vertebra.
   f Joint contractures can be prevented by correct positioning of limbs, putting the joints through a range of movements, and controlling spasms.

g Tetraplegic patients can experience sweating attacks.
h A patient with a high lesion will require urgent treatment of an upper respiratory tract infection.
i Tetraplegic and paraplegic patients have to give up the idea of having any meaningful sex life with their partners.
j Tetraplegic patients may be able to drive cars which are specially adapted.

4 *Answer the following question*

James Wilson is a 28-year-old paraplegic patient who has been admitted to your ward via the casualty department and is to be taken to theatre for a laparotomy.

What are the important considerations of the admission interview? Describe the management of Mr Wilson during the postoperative period following removal of the appendix.

■ Answers

1 *a* Surgical excision of the lamina of the vertebra frequently performed to relieve the symptoms of a slipped disc.
b Slipped disc. The nucleus pulposus of the disc protrudes through a weakened or ruptured annulus fibrosus.
c Paralysis from the waist down.
d Paralysis involving all four limbs and the trunk.
e A bladder with weak muscle power and no reflex activity. May be emptied by manual compression.
f Electronic devices and electromechanical equipment. Devices are usually easy to operate and designed to suit the ability of individual patients, e.g. suck and blow mechanisms for operating wheelchairs.
g A collection of dead tissue.
h Incising the muscles of a sphincter usually the urethra.
i The amount of urine left in the bladder following the act of micturition.
j Contraction of anal sphincter when skin around the anal region is touched.

2 *a* It takes approximately 4–6 weeks for the body to recover from spinal shock. In the days following injury wasting of the tissues and trophic skin changes may appear rapidly.
b The fracture is reduced by appropriately positioning the patient on pillows.
c Because, unfortunately, if the patient is allowed to develop one complication this can lead to a variety of others, e.g. pressure sores, contractures, spasms, bladder problems, urinary infection and so on.

d A spasm is the involuntary movement of muscle, so that a patient whose limbs are paralysed may experience erratic movements of the limbs which are beyond his control. A full bladder or bowel may give rise to spasms. The pathway to the brain is interrupted by damage to the cord so that reflexes are at a spinal level and movements are not co-ordinated by the brain. They can be very distressing for the patient and can be caused by contractures which means that joints may become stiff and held in a particular position, so that shortening of muscles in this way has to be prevented by physiotherapy and eventually continued by the patient himself.

3 *a* False
   b True
   c False
   d True
   e False
   f True
   g True
   h True
   i False
   j True.

4 You should consider including the following points in your answer:
   a Establish how long he has been a paraplegic. (He will be able to tell you the level of the lesion.) Establish his pattern of living, i.e. does he empty bowels in the morning or evening? Does he take apperients/suppositories, etc? What time does he get up in the morning and exactly in what order are things like bathing, toileting and dressing done? Establish how he manages his bladder. Find out how he places his pillows in bed and how often he turns himself. Has he brought a mirror with him to check his skin? Will he need waking in the night so that he can turn himself, so that the night nurses may be informed? (Other patients will not appreciate an alarm clock at 3/4-hourly intervals.)

Note how the patient himself is feeling and his complaints.

The amount of information gained at this time will obviously depend on the patient's condition but it is important to establish a rapport with the patient, and he may be particularly frightened of being in a general hospital as opposed to a spinal unit. The main consideration apart from that given to his general condition is for him to be reassured that his routine as far as possible will be maintained and that the nurses recognize that he, probably better than anybody, knows how to care for himself as far as the daily living activities are concerned.

b Ensure that vital observations are monitored at frequent regular intervals.
Observation of the wound dressing.
Maintenance and care of intravenous therapy and fluid balance.
Observe urinary output.
Maintain correct position in bed and carry out frequent regular turns. A chart should be used for this purpose until such time as the patient is able to resume responsibility for turning himself.
Care of the urinary appliances will be assumed by the nurses until the patient is able.
Observations of the skin regularly.
Patients may be given a wash of the hands and face a few hours following surgery. A mouthwash can be given at the same time and the patient gradually raised in the bed by giving him a few extra pillows.
The patient may require analgesia postoperatively. The immediate postoperative care and resumption of fluids and diet are as for any other surgical patient. Thereafter attention will have to be given to the equipment the patient may require to get in and out of bed, e.g. monkey pole and preferably his own wheelchair. He should be closely supervized and assisted when he gets out of bed for the first few days following surgery. Consideration should be given to the bathroom and toilet area (he may require to spend some time in the toilet – so the provision of an inflatable rubber seat would be useful). Depending on the type of urinary appliance he may require facilities for their washing. Alternatively the disposable variety may be supplied while he is in hospital. The patient would in all probability be very willing to adapt to his surroundings provided he is involved in discussions regarding his care and the facilities that are available.

Arrangements can be made with relatives to bring in the patient's clothes as he may prefer to get dressed once he is able to spend much of the day up. Rests can be taken by lying on the bed for periodic intervals during the course of the day, and pillows placed appropriately. Should problems arise in relation to his paraplegia the nearest spinal injury unit may be contacted.

Following removal of the sutures arrangements are made for the patient to be discharged home and an appointment made for him to be followed up by the surgeon in the outpatient department.

□ Comment

Students in general training do not have much opportunity for nursing a patient who has sustained spinal cord injury. The purpose of this kind of question is not to test her ability in caring for the acute spinal injury patient as much as to test her awareness of his needs, possible difficulties, and the kind of rigorous rehabilitation programme he has undergone.

5 Joints

The objectives of this chapter are to:
1 Describe briefly the structure and function of joints.
2 Describe the management of a patient admitted to the orthopaedic unit for a meniscectomy.
3 Describe the treatment and management of patients with rheumatoid arthritis and osteoarthritis.
4 State the principles of the nursing management of the patient following surgery of the hip.

■ JOINTS

A joint is formed where two or more bones come together. Joints are classified as:
a fibrous (immovable) – sutures of the skull.
b cartilaginous (slightly movable).
  i primary – e.g. epiphysis.
  ii secondary (between vertebral bodies).
c synovial (freely movable), e.g. hip joint.

Joints are so designed that where movement is desirable they are freely movable (synovial) and in those parts of the body where free movement is not so desirable they are restricted in their movements, i.e. slightly movable or immovable.

The structure and function of joints is effected by the shape of bones coming together and by the surrounding soft tissue structures and skeletal muscle. Skeletal muscles are also called striped or voluntary muscles and receive their nerve supply via the cranial and spinal nerves. Muscles require and receive a good blood supply which enters the muscle with the nerves at the neurovascular hilum. Muscles work in groups to bring about a given movement by means of prime movers and antagonists, e.g. the quadriceps will *extend* the knee while the hamstrings are relaxed; conversely, the hamstrings will *flex* the knee while the quadriceps relax. Muscles are attached to bones at two points; while the nerve supply is intact muscles remain in a state of tone.

Freely movable joints (synovial)

Those joints which are freely movable are found where much movement is required in order to be able to function effectively.

Each joint is enclosed in a capsule (fibrous tissue). The smoothness of the joint is provided by articular cartilage on the bone ends and the synovial membrane lining the remainder of the joint. This secretes small amounts of synovial fluid which serves to lubricate the joint surfaces. Synovial joints may be described as:

☐ *a Ball and socket – movements include:*
flexion/extension
abduction/adduction
rotation
circumduction

The shoulder and the hip are ball and socket joints.

☐ *b Hinge – movements include:*
flexion/extension

The interphalangeal joints and the elbow are examples of hinge joints.

☐ *c Condyloid – movements include:*
flexion/extension
abduction/adduction

The wrist is an example of a condyloid joint.

☐ *d Plane*
This joint allows gliding movements only between the surfaces of adjoining bones. Examples are found between the bones of the tarsus and carpus.

☐ *e Pivot*
This allows rotation movement which takes place at the superior radio-ulnar joint to allow pronation and supination of the forearm.

MENISCECTOMY

The knee joint (Fig. 10) is a modified hinge joint allowing flexion and extension with slight rotation when the knee is flexed. Its stability rests largely on good support provided by the quadriceps muscles. Hence, the importance of isometric quadriceps exercise following meniscectomy. The joint is made up of the femoral condyles articulating with the upper end of the tibia. The cruciate ligaments serve to hold the femur and tibia together and provide further stability of the joint. Movement of the femoral

Joints 61

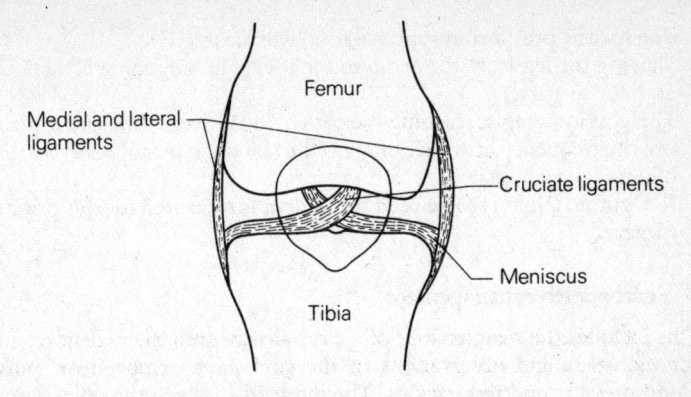

Fig. 10 The knee joint (schematic)

condyles on the tibia are facilitated by the presence of the menisci (semilunar cartilages) – medial and lateral. Further stability of the joint is provided by the strong medial and lateral ligaments which are extra-capsular.

Synovial membrane lines the interior of the joint extensively and there are synovial bursae around the knee joint. The patella is situated anteriorly.

- **Injuries to the semilunar cartilages**

The cartilage on the medial side is most often affected because it is attached to the medial ligament. The injury is often caused by a rotation movement while weight-bearing. The patient complains of pain and locking of the knee joint which may be accompanied by swelling. The problem may be rectified by manipulation, but if it is recurring it may require operative treatment to remove the cartilage (meniscectomy).

- **Pre-operative preparation** (meniscectomy)

The patients are more commonly male and are usually fit and healthy on admission. The patient will be given a physical examination by the doctor who will also take a history. Blood will be obtained for a full blood count including haemoglobin estimations, a chest radiograph prior to general anaesthesia, as well as radiological examination of the knee if not already done. The surgeon will explain the procedure to the patient and obtain the necessary consent for surgery.

The specific pre-operative preparation will include:
a Shaving the leg from the groin to the toe. (The surgeon will mark the limb for surgery.)
b The physiotherapist teaching the patient 'quadriceps drill' and explaining the frequency at which they need to be done postoperatively (five minutes every hour).
c If a 'gutter splint' is to be used the patient is measured for this prior to surgery.

■ Postoperative management

This includes the maintenance of a clear airway until the patient regains consciousness and observations of the vital signs, temperature, pulse, blood pressure and respirations. The intervals at which the observations are made are increased as the patient's condition stabilizes and improves. Analgesia will be required in the immediate postoperative period.

The knee is usually covered with a dressing underneath a Robert Jones' bandage (pressure bandage). The limb may or may not be supported by a gutter splint. The limb is placed on a pillow lengthwise. As soon as the patient regains consciousness and vital signs are stable he is gradually sat up and commences quadriceps drill. Regular and frequent observation is made of the circulation, mobility and sensation to toes.

The pressure bandage is usually retained until the sutures are removed in about 10 days. The patient may be allowed up after a few days or not until the sutures are removed depending on the particular surgeon. Similarly, the patient may be allowed to weight-bear at once or wait. If he is to be non-weight-bearing this can be achieved by the use of a wheelchair or crutches which the patient is taught to use.

Provided there is no effusion of the joint when the sutures are removed, the patient may take weight through the leg, initially under the supervision of the physiotherapist, and be re-educated in heel-to-toe walking unless he has been allowed to weight-bear immediately postoperatively. The patient is reviewed by the orthopaedic surgeon in the outpatient department and will be advised regarding return to work and resumption of sporting activities.

■ RHEUMATOID ARTHRITIS

This is a disorder that is often treated by a team of doctors including a rheumatologist as well as the orthopaedic surgeon. The disease process is not confined to joints and patients are frequently systemically ill. Rheumatoid arthritis occurs more frequently in women than men and the cause of the disease is not known. It may be that both genetic and environmental factors play a part in the development of the condition. It is also thought that it may be due to a defect in the patient's immune system. The rheumatoid factor has been found to be present in a high percentage of patients with rheumatoid arthritis.

The condition can arise at any age but most commonly between the ages of 35 and 55 years. Although the disease in its onset is usually slow and progressive, a few patients may suffer a sudden onset with rise in temperature accompanied by pain in the joints. Others, however, may simply complain of tiredness and vague joint and muscular stiffness and possible pain for some time before there is obvious disorder of the joints. More commonly rheumatoid arthritis tends to develop in the smaller joints and is symmetrical in distribution, i.e. it may start in the fingers and spread to the wrists and elbows, and so on. Any synovial joint may be affected.

■ The joints

Changes in the joints include swelling and proliferation of the synovial membrane. Eventually this thickening process of the synovial membrane spreads and causes destruction of the articular cartilage by enzymes. As the disease progresses the joints may be gradually destroyed by the fibrous tissue and ankylosis. Movement is limited, deformity and muscle wasting become apparent. Nodules may also be present beneath the skin.

Rheumatoid arthritis is a progressive disease for which, as yet, there is no cure. The patient experiences acute attacks relieved by periods of remission. The course of the disease varies from patient to patient. Although the main feature of the disease is the joint involvement, when the patient is admitted to hospital during an acute attack he is usually feeling ill and will be seen to have a low-grade pyrexia and tachycardia. He may be feeling unwell generally with tiredness, loss of appetite and weight. The joints may be swollen, stiff and painful and the patient reluctant to move them. Lymph nodes may be enlarged and the blood picture shows a raised ESR, leucocytosis and anaemia.

■ Investigations

These include:

Radiological examination of the joints.
Blood investigations, e.g. full blood count and haemoglobin estimation.

Erythrocyte sedimentation rate (ESR).
Estimation of plasma proteins (increase in globulin and fibrinogen).
Rheumatoid factor tests, e.g. Rose-Waaler test, latex-fixation test.
Synovial fluid. Examination of the synovial fluid may also be ordered.

■ Treatment

This is aimed at relieving the symptoms, to prevent/correct joint deformity, to improve the general health of the patient so that as much independence as possible is retained. Drugs which may be used include analgesics and anti-inflammatory drugs, e.g. antimalarial, gold, and corticosteroids. All these drugs have possible side-effects and the patient's reaction to therapy must be closely supervised and monitored. Anaemia is treated appropriately. Corticosteroids may also be injected directly into a joint (intra-articular) by the doctor.

Surgical treatment may be required for the joints and this may include synovectomy, arthrodesis and arthroplasty. Silastic implants are now available for the smaller joints of the hands.

■ Nursing management of the patient admitted to hospital with an acute exacerbation of the disease

□ *Placement in the ward*

On admission into hospital the patient will be feeling ill and be in considerable pain. Consideration should therefore be given to placing the patient in that part of the ward where maximum rest and quiet will be achieved.

□ *Position in bed*

The patient should be placed in a clean warm bed with a firm, hard base. He may initially adopt the position in which he is most comfortable, adequately supported with pillows. However, the patient's position will have to be changed at intervals to prevent sore formation and joint contractures. Splintage may be ordered to maintain optimum functional positions of affected limbs and to provide a means of resting the painful joints in the acute phase. A cradle should be placed to protect the limbs from the weight of the bedclothes, and a full-length sheepskin beneath the patient may be useful.

□ *Skin and general hygiene*

Close attention is required of the patient's skin and nurses should regularly look at all those areas prone to pressure sore formation. Any change in the skin which may occur as a result of vasculitis should also be noted. Initially the patient may require washing and bed bathing by the nurses. Splints are removed for washing and care must be taken in handling the limbs, not only because of pain experienced by the patient but also the tendency of rheumatoid joints to dislocate. The affected joints may require complete rest during the acute illness in which case a plaster of Paris cast may be applied for 2–3 weeks. Frequent washes may be required while the patient is pyrexial. Sweating may also be present, particularly on the palms of the hands and soles of the feet. The hair should be kept clean and styled as the patient wishes. This will have to be done for the patient initially. Care must be taken of the nails which may be brittle and special attention paid to the eyes as the patient may complain of dryness. Any abnormalities found during the course of washing the patient should be reported to the doctor. The patient's teeth must be cleaned and mouthwashes offered at intervals.

□ *Mobility*

While rest must be achieved for the patient both generally and locally he must be moved gently and his position changed at regular intervals to prevent sores developing. Change from the semi-recumbent position to lying with one pillow should also be made during the course of the day so that the hip and knee joints may be stretched. The physiotherapist will visit the patient regularly and carry out an assessment. Specific physiotherapy to the joints affected will range from passive, active assisted to active exercises which the patient can practise throughout the day. When muscle power is adequate the patient may bear weight (if the weight-bearing joints are affected).

Heat treatment may be applied by the physiotherapist prior to exercise in the form of wax, hydropacks, or infra-red irradiation. A hydrotherapy pool is useful and can be used for exercises. The occupational therapist will also be involved in assessing the patient's ability to perform daily living activities. As the patient's mobility improves he will be able to do more for himself with less assistance from the nurses.

□ *Eating and drinking*

As with cleaning the teeth the patient will initially have to be helped with eating. It is not very pleasant for patients to have to be fed and much sensitivity is required on the part of the nurse. As soon as the patient's condition improves assistance, such as cutting up meat and the use of non-slip mats and adapted cutlery, will ensure that the patient can manage meals himself which will do much in the way of restoring independence and help the patient to realize that progress is being made. Fluids should be encouraged and the use of suitable cups will enable the patient to take fluids himself. Fluids should be poured for the patient until such time that he can do so himself which may be achieved earlier if the jug on the locker is only half filled and therefore lighter in weight. Initially the diet should be light and well balanced. Adequate intake of calcium and proteins can be achieved by providing milk drinks for the patient. Any nausea or vomiting should be reported; this may be caused by the drug therapy.

The occupational therapist will assess the patient and supply any aids or adaptations to enable the patient gain independence in eating and drinking.

□ *Elimination*

The urine is tested on admission. The patient will require help with elimination initially and a female urinal may be more convenient than a bedpan and less strenuous for the patient. The genital region will have to be washed by the nurses until the patient is able to do this for himself. Constipation should be avoided and the doctor may prescribe a mild aperient to keep the bowels regular. Care of the anal region will be the nurse's responsibility until the patient is able to clean himself. Bedpans may be discarded for the commode or sanichair as the patient's condition improves. This is usually welcomed by the patient.

□ *Rest and sleep*

It is important to achieve mental as well as physical rest. Cheerful but quietly pleasant surroundings for the patient with sufficient room for flowers, plants, photographs, etc., without cluttering the space required by the patient. Time spent arranging the pillows with the patient before he settles down for the night is worth while, for an irritating discomfort can delay the onset of sleep. Books, television and newspapers may help to give him the degree of activity he requires during the day without exhausting him so that a good night's sleep may be achieved. The doctor may prescribe sedation if the patient is unable to sleep at night. During the day exercise periods and nursing care should be organized so that adequate rest periods are also provided. A balance between rest, activity and sleep must be found to suit each patient.

□ *Communication*

Relatives, as always, should be fully informed of the patient's progress. Their understanding of the need for rest is also important so that they can arrange their visiting times with this in mind. A female patient should be given adequate help with make-up which she may want to wear before visitors arrive. If she generally wears make-up this should be encouraged. Relatives should feel that they can talk to the nurses, who should make themselves available and approachable at any time. Some of the deformities in rheumatoid arthritis can be quite severe and obvious to others, so patients may be concerned about deformities of the hands, overriding of the fingers, swelling of the knuckles and ulnar deviation. A woman may no longer be able to manicure her nails as she likes them, and so on. While in hospital the nurse can help with these activities which may be very important to the patient, and when at home, a relative, friend or neighbour may continue the assistance.

Assessment of the patient and her ability to manage at home is made in the light of communication with all disciplines concerned: physiotherapist, occupational therapist, medical social worker, and in the case of occupational problems the disablement resettlement officer (DRO). Full discussions must be held with all concerned including the patient and relatives. Continuing assessment, facilities, aids and home alterations may have to be made as the needs of the patient alter as the disease progresses.

■ OSTEOARTHRITIS

This is a slowly progressive arthritis which differs from rheumatoid arthritis in that the patients are usually in good health and may be overweight. It differs also in its tendency to affect mainly the larger weight-bearing joints, often one at a time and the age-group of the patients tends to be older. Osteoarthritis can be referred to as *primary* when the cause of the disorder is not apparent and genetics, occupation, weight and age of the patient are considered contributory factors. *Secondary* osteoarthritis may develop as a result of a faulty joint mechanism following, for example, congenital abnormality or previous trauma.

Initial degeneration takes place in the articular cartilage at the point where maximum weight is borne so that the underlying bone is exposed, and eventually hardens, and becomes dense with a shiny surface (eburnation). Small outgrowths of bone develop at the edges of the articular cartilage (osteophytes). Excess synovial membrane becomes fibrosed as eventually does the joint capsule, giving rise to contracture and limited movement.

Signs and symptoms of osteoarthritis are generally confined to the affected joint and arise gradually. Initially there may be some aching of the joint following use which may eventually become painful. The pain is usually relieved by rest, but following a rest period the joint becomes stiff. As the disease develops, pain may become more apparent and difficult to cope with when sleep is disturbed. Restriction of movement becomes more obvious and stiffness leads to deformity of the joint. Grating sounds may be felt in the joint or sometimes heard. There may also be effusion of the joint.

Radiological examination of the affected joint will be requested.

■ Treatment

Treatment is directed towards relieving pain, correction or prevention of deformity and maintaining or restoring the function of the affected joint. Initially this may be achieved by the patient's losing weight if he is obese, and avoiding undue strain on the affected joint. Advice is given to the patient regarding rest periods during the day as this is an important part of treatment. Exercises to restore the muscle tone will be taught by the physiotherapist. Postural exercises may be required and heat in varying forms, e.g. short wave diathermy, infra-red, may prove beneficial. Analgesic drugs such as aspirin (which may be enteric coated) may be prescribed for the relief of pain. Other anti-inflammatory drugs such as indomethacin may be helpful but such drugs do have possible serious side-effects and are only prescribed under close supervision of the patient. Aids such as raised shoes or a walking stick may also help to relieve stress on the joint. These measures can help the patient and minimize pain and development of deformity for a number of years, but there may come a time when the patient has to consider changing his occupation.

Surgical intervention may need to be considered at some time. The surgeon will consider many factors and discuss these with the patient in determining the surgery which is most appropriate for that individual. Surgical procedures include arthrodesis, osteotomy and arthroplasty (joint replacement). Factors such as age, severity of the arthritis, movement of other joints, the patient's occupation, and so on, will be considered.

□ *Osteotomy* (Fig. 11)

This procedure may be used in the early treatment of osteoarthritis of the hip joint to alter the line of weight-bearing. It involves the division of the bone followed by the correction of the deformity. The correction once achieved is then splinted to maintain the position.

Upper tibial osteotomy may be performed for osteoarthritis of the knee joint.

□ *Arthrodesis*

This is the term used to describe surgical fusion of a joint. Indications are pain and instability of a joint and, in some situations, following the failure of joint replacement. Nowadays it is carried out much less often.

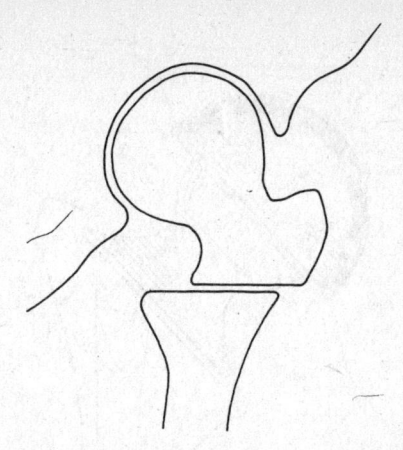

Fig. 11 Osteotomy

☐ *Arthroplasty* (joint replacement)
This is a surgical procedure performed to refashion a joint. Nowadays joint replacement is the preferred term. In the *hip joint* the following methods may be encountered. There are numerous named types by which the joint itself may be replaced and the nurse should apprise herself of the type(s) used in her own hospital.
1 Total hip replacement (Fig. 12).
2 Replacement of the femoral head (Fig. 13).
3 Cup arthroplasty, i.e. a Vitallium cup in the acetabulum to contain the femoral head.
4 Excision of the femoral head and neck (Girdlestone). This is only done as a salvage procedure when other methods have failed.
   The knee joint can also be totally replaced by an artificial joint.
   Apart from the weight-bearing joints already mentioned osteoarthritis also affects the spine, where the operative treatment may be a spinal fusion; less commonly seen is osteoarthritis of the upper limbs where treatment may be conservative or surgical.

■ **Management of a patient following surgery on the hip joint**

Nursing the patient following surgery of the hip joint often causes confusion for the learner because of the variety of operations, the different

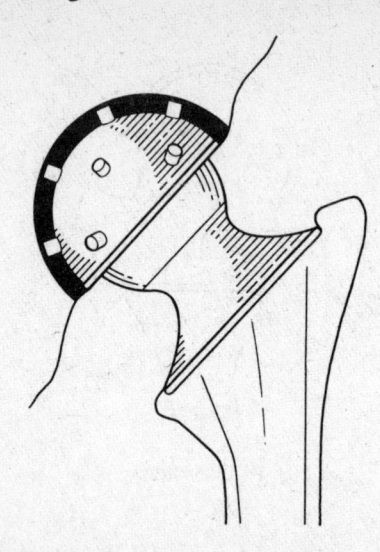

Fig. 12 Total hip replacement – McKee-Farrar

types of prosthesis that are available, and after-care which varies with different surgeons who have their own preferred methods. It is therefore of the utmost importance that nurses familiarize themselves with these variances in procedure, always checking with the person in charge of the ward about moving a patient in any particular way, and what positions are to be avoided. There are certain fundamental points which are worthy of consideration.

The pre-operative management of the patient is as for any major surgical procedure, and the surgeon will explain the type of surgery to the patient and give him some idea of how long it will be before he is up and walking again. The physiotherapist will visit the patient and explain to him the kinds of movement to carry out postoperatively as well as those to be avoided; exercises to be practised will also be taught.

□ *Postoperative management*

Postoperatively the usual management of the patient is carried out including observations of the vital signs, temperature, pulse, blood pressure and respiratory rate. The dressing and any drains are observed for signs of haemorrhage. A blood transfusion may be in progress on his return to the ward. On completion, hydration may be maintained for a few hours by

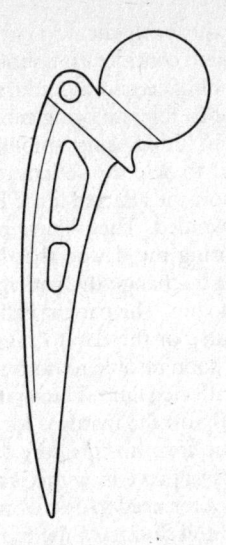

Fig. 13 Austin Moore prosthesis for the replacement of femoral head

intravenous therapy, until such time as the patient is taking fluids orally, a light diet is usually tolerated the following day. A weight-reducing diet may be given if the patient is obese and has not lost weight prior to surgery. Analgesia should be given to control the pain postoperatively and a record made of the patient's urinary output.

The patient returns to the ward in the recumbent position and the limbs are maintained in a position of abduction by means of a wedge between the limbs or in some instances a large triangular pillow may be used. Very occasionally, the patient may return to the ward with traction applied to the affected limb.

□ *Mobilization*
As the patient's condition improves and the vital signs are stable he is placed in the semi-recumbent position supported by pillows. The patient is *not* sat fully upright as this allows flexion of the hip joint. In some units a pillow is placed lengthwise under the affected limb (from the knee down) so as to clear the heel off the bed. The heel on the affected side must be closely observed. Lifting the patient on and off bedpans is done with adequate numbers of nurses. At least three nurses will be required – two to lift, one to place and remove the bedpan – until the patient is able to help

by using a monkey pole, probably the next day. The doctor will prescribe analgesia for the patient and consideration should be given to the time it is given and the carrying out of certain procedures in relation to this so that the patient is better able to tolerate being moved, and so on. When the patient is able to help with lifting using a monkey pole the *unaffected* limb may be flexed at the knee to help the patient to raise himself, but a nurse will be required to support the affected limb. Full flexion and rotation of the hip joint must be avoided. The pillows behind the patient may be removed for periods during the day so that he may assume the supine position. This will serve to change the patient's position and avoid any flexion contracture of the hip. The patient will require lifting at frequent intervals during the course of the day to relieve pressure on the sacral region. The patient will soon be able to do this himself with the aid of a monkey pole and the unaffected limb. The lift itself need only be sufficient to ease the patient slightly off the mattress for a few seconds, enough to relieve the pressure on the area. It is pressure that causes sores to develop and the only effective way of preventing this is to relieve the pressure. The patient should be aware of the need to do this and also the need to prevent rotation of the limb and full flexion of the hip joint because the femoral head can dislocate.

Deep breathing and leg exercises, as taught pre-operatively, will be encouraged. These include quadriceps drill, active movements of the feet and toes and gluteal contractions.

It is usually the physiotherapist who helps the patient out of bed initially, at the same time maintaining abduction and avoiding too much flexion at the hip joint. Great care is taken when the patient stands for the first time as he may feel dizzy. When the patient eventually progresses as far as sitting out in a chair, the chair should be carefully selected so that it is reasonably high. The physiotherapist will teach the patient how to lower himself into the chair and rise again. By this time the patient will be able to use the toilet and special aids are available for the purpose of raising the height of the toilet seat, again, to avoid excessive flexion of the hip. The physiotherapist will also select the most appropriate walking aid for the patient.

Age of the patient, previous mobility and the type of surgery will determine to what extent and how quickly the patient progresses. The programme designed by the physiotherapist will take all the factors into account including the patient's home situation. The occupational therapist will assess the patient regarding aids that may be required for dressing, such as help with stockings and shoes. The patient is advised to bring a comfortable low heel supportive pair of shoes into hospital with him, alternatively the relatives may bring them in later.

Nurses do not have the same in-depth knowledge possessed by physiotherapists, but it is helpful for them to be aware of the types of exercises that the physiotherapist performs and expects of the patient. They must be aware of those movements which it is important to avoid: *flexion* and *rotation*. They should understand the progressive nature of the physiotherapy, which is within each patient's capacity. Some patients are up standing on the second or third day following hip surgery (depending on the type) while others will remain in bed for longer periods – perhaps on traction, but the principles of immobilization and ambulation will still apply, i.e. appropriate exercise in bed, prevention of flexion and rotation deformities, to gradual weight-bearing, sitting correctly, through to walking.

The patient will require some help in getting in and out of the bath for the first few times. Before being discharged he is advised about resting for periods during the day, i.e. lying on the bed, the amount of walking and so on. The patient may continue to attend the physiotherapy department as an outpatient. He will be reviewed by the surgeon in the outpatient department as long as the surgeon considers this to be necessary.

■ THE NORWICH CEMENTLESS TOTAL HIP REPLACEMENT

Recently, this new total hip replacement has been added to the other types which are available, some of which have been discussed in previous pages.

■ The reasons for failure of cemented hip replacement operations

1 Implant design failure.
2 Articulating surface failure.
3 Interface failure.

■ Principles of the Norwich hip system

1 To transfer adequate load to the proximal femur and avoid stress protection.
2 To provide, by simple instrumentation, a perfect interference fit for initial fixation.
3 To provide a stable benign interface between implant and bone or fibrous tissue.

4 To correct soft tissue contracture.
5 To equalize leg length.
6 To allow easy revision.

The hip system has been designed to overcome the shortcomings of available hip implants, and to provide a safe alternative to cement fixation particularly in the younger patient. The overall philosophy aims to re-establish normal load bearing transfer between the pelvis and the femur. Proximal load bearing, the essence of a successful hip implant, is encouraged for the first time by accurate instrumentation and good design. Success on the femoral side is dependent upon calcar loading which in turn is very sensitive to the following parameters: implant design, instrumentation and surgical technique. Careful assessment of the pathological anatomy and skeletal geometry in the individual case, together with the provision of many sizes of implant for both the acetabular and femoral sides guarantees a perfect interference fit with bone without the use of acrylic cement. Placing the implant into an anatomical position encourages leg length equality and identifies correctable soft tissue contracture.

■ Indications and contra-indications

The usual clinical principles which govern patient selection apply when using a Norwich cementless component. The system may be used when the surgeon considers that a cemented implant would be likely to fail during the lifetime of the patient, and may be offered as an alternative procedure for patients who might otherwise be considered for proximal femoral osteotomy or arthrodesis.

The Norwich components have been used in osteoarthritis, rheumatoid disease, avascular necrosis, post-traumatic arthritis, non-union of femoral neck fracture, and in revision arthroplasty where there is adequate recipient bone.

Caution is advised when offering Norwich uncemented components to patients with osteoporosis and where bone remodelling is compromised by the use of steroids and possibly anti-inflammatory agents. The use of Norwich cementless components is contra-indicated in the presence of infection, where there is poor bone quality and when the patient may not or cannot comply with the advised postoperative regime.

■ After-care

The initial after-care of the patient does not differ from convention. The patient remains in bed for 3–7 days. The physiotherapist supervises range of movement exercises within the limits of any dislocatable hip during this early period. When walking with elbow crutches only 15kg of weight as measured on scales is allowed to pass through the operated limb using elbow crutches at all times. This gait pattern is maintained for 3 months.

A further course of physiotherapy is often indicated when the walking aids are discarded and is directed towards strengthening muscles, particularly the glutei, and education of the patient to produce a more normal pattern of gait.

■ PRACTICE QUESTIONS

1 *What is meant by the following terms?*
   a Immovable joint
   b Synovial joint
   c Prime mover
   d Antagonists
   e Flexion
   f Extension
   g Abduction
   h Adduction
   i External rotation
   j Meniscectomy
   k Cruciate ligaments
   l Joint effusion
   m Rheumatoid arthritis
   n Synovial fluid
   o Osteophytes
   p Osteotomy
   q Osteoarthritis
   r Arthrodesis
   s Arthroplasty
   t Joint capsule.
2 *Briefly explain the following:*
   a The importance of isometric (static) quadriceps exercises following a meniscectomy, or any surgery on the knee joint.
   b Why the urine should be tested regularly for a patient with rheumatoid arthritis who is receiving a preparation of gold salts as part of the therapy.
   c Why an overweight patient with osteoarthritis is encouraged to lose weight.

d Why an osteotomy is thought to be effective for some patients with osteoarthritis.
e The functions of the semilunar cartilages (menisci) in the knee joint.

■ Answers

1 *a* An immovable joint is one that does not allow movement between the bones and is fibrous in structure.
  b A freely movable joint enclosed in a joint capsule. The surfaces of the joint are lined by synovial membrane and a small amount of synovial fluid lubricates the joint.
  c The muscles that contract in order to bring about a particular movement.
  d The muscles that bring about the opposite movement to the prime movers.
  e Flexion refers to the bending of a limb or a part of the body.
  f Extension refers to straightening the limb or a part of the body.
  g Movement where a part is moved away from the midline of the body.
  h Movement where a part is moved towards the midline of the body.
  i The rolling of a limb outwards.
  j Removal of a semilunar cartilage (meniscus) in the knee joint.
  k Ligaments found in the knee joint which help to give it stability and hold the femur and tibia together.
  l Accumulation of fluid in a joint.
  m A non-suppurative inflammatory condition affecting primarily the joints, but accompanied by systemic disturbances.
  n Fluid secreted by synovial membrane which serves to lubricate a joint.
  o Outgrowths of bone.
  p The cutting of a bone surgically.
  q A painful degenerative disease of the joints.
  r Surgical fixation of a joint which was previously movable.
  s Refashioning of a joint.
  t Fibrous tissue which encloses synovial joints.
2 *a* To maintain good tone in the quadriceps, muscles which are important to the stability of the knee joint.
  b Gold salts have many toxic reactions including nephritis.
  c Apart from the effects of obesity on the general health of the patient, the excess weight places extra strain on weight-bearing joints in particular.

d It is thought that altering the line of weight-bearing reduces the pain experienced by the patient.
e They allow the femoral condyles to fit the tibial surfaces closely and act as shock absorbers.

6 Diseases affecting bone

The objectives of this section are to:
1 Describe the condition osteomyelitis and the nursing management of a patient suffering from it.
2 Describe the nursing management of a patient with tuberculosis of the bone.
3 Outline briefly the management of bone tumours.
4 To describe the condition rickets.

■ OSTEOMYELITIS

This term describes a condition of the bone when it is infected. The disease can be blood-borne, that is, the organisms reach the bone via the bloodstream, or the organisms reach the bone directly through a wound or a skin condition such as a boil. Among the frequent causative organisms are *Staphylococcus aureus*, *Streptococcus* and *Pneumococcus*. Osteomyelitis is more frequently seen in children.

When the bone becomes infected the blood supply is affected giving rise to necrosis. Pus may subsequently spread through the Haversian canals. An abscess may develop beneath the periosteum lifting it off the bone, further depriving it of blood. The infection may spread to a neighbouring joint giving rise to septic arthritis. The abscess may burst through the overlying skin, or spread to the bone marrow. As the disease progresses sequestra may form. A new layer of bone may then surround the sequestra which is known as the involucrum.

■ Management of acute osteomyelitis

When the patient is admitted to the ward with osteomyelitis, he is usually very ill. Apart from a limb that is very painful, tender, and possibly swollen and warm to touch, the child is pyrexial with a tachycardia. Other signs may include nausea, vomiting, dry mouth and dehydration.

□ *Investigations*
a A full blood count.
b Erythrocyte sedimentation rate (ESR).

c Blood culture.
d Radiological examination of the affected part. (In the acute phase radiographs appear normal.)

Treatment consists of rest and general and local antibiotic therapy. Surgical intervention may be required. (Systemic antibiotics may be given intravenously initially.)

■ Nursing care of a child admitted with osteomyelitis

□ *Position in the ward*

When the child is admitted to hospital he should be placed in an area where maximum rest can be achieved. A side-room may be desirable for the first few days so that he is away from the main activities of the ward.

□ *Position in bed and mobilization*

The bed should have a firm base and a cradle to keep the bed clothes from resting on the affected part. The child will be allowed to assume the position in which he is most comfortable and a splint or plaster shell may be ordered to immobilize and rest the affected limb. For the first few days the nurses will have to change the child's position frequently to avoid the development of pressure sores; as his general condition improves he will be able to help himself more. Each time the child is moved care must be taken in handling the splinted limb as much pain is experienced.

□ *Observations*

The temperature, pulse and respiration are observed at frequent intervals depending on the child's condition. Any rigors are noted and reported to the doctor. (They may be indicative of complications such as joint involvement. Observations must also be made of an abnormal position of the limbs or limited mobility in a joint.)

□ *Eating and drinking*

Because he is febrile the child is unlikely to feel like eating or drinking. Maintenance of fluid balance is extremely important and, in the event of the child's not being able to tolerate sufficient oral fluids, an intravenous infusion will be set up. Intravenous fluids are then administered as prescribed by the doctor, recorded, and the infusion site observed. The nurse should find out what the child's favourite drinks are so that they can be provided and the amounts given gradually increased. Initially the diet should be light and as the condition improves a nourishing well-balanced diet will be tolerated.

□ *Skin and general hygiene*

Care should be taken of the skin and frequent observations of the pressure areas made. A blanket bath is given once a day supplemented by frequent washes of the hands and face. Tepid sponging may be used to help alleviate the pyrexia, and frequent change of bed linen because of the perspiration. A fan may be used to keep the child cool. Damp cool pads to the forehead may help to relieve headache. Every effort should be made to keep the mouth clean and moist. The child is encouraged to clean his teeth in the mornings and evenings and mouthwashes may be given at frequent intervals during the course of the day. Stimulation of saliva may be helped by giving the child boiled sweets to suck.

The nails should be kept short and clean.

☐ *Drug therapy*

Specific drug therapy includes the administration of large doses of antibiotics either intravenously or intramuscularly. These are usually continued for some time after the acute phase has subsided.

A drug such as paracetamol (Panadol) (there is a paediatric version, Paracetamol Elixir Paediatric) may be prescribed to help reduce the temperature and relieve the pain.

Blood transfusions may be required for the treatment of any anaemia which may be present.

☐ *Elimination*

Urine On admission to the ward a specimen of urine is obtained and tested. Urinary output should be observed and recorded on the fluid balance chart. Careful lifting on and off bedpans will be required and pillows used to provide support as necessary.

Bowels Constipation should be avoided; the use of suppositories may be necessary should the child become constipated. The nurse should ensure privacy for the use of a bedpan and give help with cleaning following its use.

☐ *Communication*

The parents should be kept informed at all times regarding the child's progress. Depending on the child's age an explanation should also be given to him regarding his condition and what is going to be done.

How much time the mother will spend with the child will depend on such things as his or her age, other children at home, the husband's hours of work, whether or not members of the family live near by. Whatever the circumstances, the support given to the parents should be appropriate. If the mother and/or father are able to spend much time with the child they may like to be involved in his management. They should also be given information regarding where the telephones are, the toilet, where they can go for a cup of tea and something to eat. Within a few days when the child is beginning to feel better and the temperature is subsiding, perhaps books and puzzles can be used to provide some activity which does not require too much effort. Children often like to have stories read to them even though they are able to read themselves.

Surgical intervention is usually considered necessary if the child does not respond fairly quickly to the above measures or if an abscess is present. The child, general condition permitting, is then prepared for theatre and the abscess drained. A period of immobilization follows. The surgeon will indicate when the child can take weight (lower limb) and begin walking again.

Osteomyelitis can become chronic when proper healing does not take place. The child's general health is poor and is subject to 'flare ups' of the condition. Operative treatment can include such things as drainage of the abscess, removal of infected material, sequestrectomy, skin grafts, osteotomies for correction of deformity. Occasionally a Brodie's abscess (this is a cavity filled with pus and surrounded by sclerosed bone) may develop. Antibiotics are also required for the treatment of chronic osteomyelitis.

■ TUBERCULOSIS OF BONE

Tuberculosis is a disease less commonly seen nowadays due to improved living conditions, hygiene, controlled milk supplies, better nutrition, improved public health services and vaccination programmes. The causative organism is the tubercle bacillus which may be the human type (that is inhaled from another person whose lungs are infected with tuberculosis) or the bovine type (when milk from infected cows is ingested). The bone or joints can become infected by tuberculosis usually following a primary focus elsewhere in the body or they may be primarily infected. The organism is spread via the lymphatic system and bloodstream.

The organism invades the bone or structures of a joint causing erosion and caseation leading to a cold abscess. Sinuses may develop.

A patient with tuberculosis will have local signs and symptoms including pain which is aggravated by movement causing spasm of muscles which may become wasted. The affected area may be hot, tender and swollen. Deformity may also be apparent. General symptoms and signs include loss of weight and appetite, feeling of tiredness and weakness. The patient may appear pale and unwell. The temperature may be raised in the evenings accompanied by 'night sweats'.

■ Investigations include

Radiological examination of the chest and affected part.

82 Orthopaedic Nursing

Blood sample – full blood count (FBC) and erythrocyte sedimentation rate (ESR).
Samples of urine and sputum should be obtained and cultured for acid fast bacilli.
Mantoux or Heaf test may be ordered.
A specimen of pus may be obtained for laboratory investigation.
A biopsy of a lymph node may also be performed.

■ Treatment

Treatment of bone tuberculosis can be divided into three categories:
1. General treatment which includes drug therapy.
2. Local treatment which may consist of immobilization of the affected joint in the position of choice.
3. Operative treatment: surgery may be necessary at some stage of the disease.

□ Drugs

The following drugs may be used in the treatment of tuberculosis: capreomycin, cycloserine, ethambutol, ethionamide, kanamycin, isoniazid, pyrazinamide, rifampicin, streptomycin.

A combination of three anti-tubercular drugs is given; it is referred to as the intensive triple drug regime.

Three drugs are given to reduce the organisms as quickly as possible. It also minimizes the chance of persistence of drug-resistance organisms. Drug therapy is prolonged because these organisms multiply slowly. The majority of patients improve rapidly once anti-tuberculosis therapy has begun.

A typical regime consists of intramuscular streptomycin together with oral ethambutol and isoniazid.

1. *Streptomycin* is given intramuscularly for either 30 or 90 days: 1 gram (g) daily for 30 days or 2–3 times a week for 90 days.
   Mode of action: Inhibits protein synthesis by direct action on ribosomes.
2. *Ethambutol* (EMB)
   15mg/kg/body-weight. Usually given as a daily single dose.
   Mode of action: Inhibits RNA synthesis and phosphate metabolism.
3. *Isoniazid* (INH)
   5mg/kg/body-weight usually given as a daily single dose.
   Mode of action: Interferes with DNA synthesis and intermediary metabolism.
   INH and EMB are continued for approximately two years.

■ Nursing care of a patient with tuberculosis of bone

□ *Position of the patient in the ward*
The patient is placed in that part of the ward where adequate ventilation is provided with access to move the bed outside if local conditions permit.

□ *Position in bed and mobilization*
This is determined by the site of the lesion; if the spine is affected the patient may be immobilized on a plaster bed. If so, it is useful for the patient to practise lying on his back in bed for long periods for a couple of days prior to being immobilized on a plaster bed. He should practise eating and drinking in this position, and using a bedpan or urinal. The use of a head mirror is an essential part of the management and the patient should get used to viewing his surroundings by using the mirror while in the supine position.

Tuberculosis of other joints requires immobilization and the degree will depend on the type of splintage or appliance used. The physiotherapist will treat the patient, teaching him deep breathing exercises and exercises for all joints not immobilized.

Change of position is carried out regularly to prevent the development of pressure sores.

□ *Eating and drinking*
Fluids should be encouraged to prevent renal complications, and a variety should be provided so that the patient does not get tired of the same drinks. In the case of a child an effort should be made not only to vary the drinks but to provide those that he particularly likes.

The food provided should be varied, attractively served and well balanced. Every effort should be made to encourage the patient to eat and steps taken to establish why meals are not being taken. The importance of diet should be discussed with the patient and the necessary degree of assistance provided. The eating of meals can become a problem particularly if the patient feels nauseous, which may occur as a result of drug therapy. Much patience and tact is therefore required of the nurse in relation to meals.

□ *Skin and personal hygiene*
The amount of help the patient will require with washing will depend on the degree of immobilization, ranging from almost total dependence through to self-care with the minimum of assistance. Observation of the skin over the pressure areas is required (this may be done using the Norton or Waterlow scale, as well as by direct observation). Any rashes noted must be reported to the surgeon as they may be a result of anti-tuberculous drugs; the application of calamine lotion may be ordered for the irritation.

Facilities should be provided for the patient to clean his own teeth. Dentures should be removed and cleaned for the patient. The hair and nails should be kept clean.

☐ *Elimination*

Urinary output should be noted and tested periodically for abnormalities. Proteinuria may result from the administration of streptomycin.

Urinals and bedpans will have to be used. Constipation should be avoided and the use of mild aperients may be required to this end. Any diarrhoea should be reported as it may be due to one or other of the prescribed drugs.

☐ *Observations*

These should be directed towards the response of the patient to therapy. Temperature and pulse should be taken at intervals and recorded. 'Night sweats' should be recorded and reported to the surgeon accordingly. The patient should be observed for the possible side-effects of drugs; streptomycin can cause damage to the auditory (VIIIth cranial) nerve so that if the patient complains of headache, ringing in the ears, giddiness, the surgeon should be informed. The patient should be observed at all times for possible complications of the disease or those of bed rest.

☐ *Rest and sleep*

Rest should be ensured for the patient. It may be that nights are disturbed because of discomfort from sweating in which case suitable rest times should be arranged during the course of the day. The fact that the patient is in bed all day does not in itself ensure adequate rest, and steps may have to be taken to ensure that this is achieved. Attention should be paid to the comfort of the patient and the rearranging of pillows may be all that is required.

☐ *Communication*

The outline of treatment should be explained to both relatives and patient. The importance of diet, sleep and rest should be discussed with them. There may be financial difficulties if the patient is the breadwinner and the help of the medical social worker may be sought.

It will be necessary to screen members of the family for tuberculosis.

■ HEALTH EDUCATION FOR BONE TUBERCULOSIS

■ Prevention of spread of infection

1 To identify, notify and effectively treat infected patients.

2 To trace the source of the infection of newly notified cases.
3 To screen the families and close contacts of newly notified cases by means of chest radiological examination (x-ray) and Mantoux testing.
4 Promote a vaccination programme for all schoolchildren at the age of 13.
5 Vaccinate newborn babies if either parent has tuberculosis.
6 Screen all immigrants coming from countries where there is known to be a high rate of tuberculosis.
7 Teach the patient and the family about the disease.
8 Some patients have other problems, e.g. alcoholism, psychiatric disorders or social problems; these patients tend to stay in hospital longer.

■ BONE TUMOURS

Like tumours elsewhere bone tumours may be benign or malignant. The former being encapsulated and contained in a particular part of the body, the latter spreading to other parts via the lymphatic system and bloodstream.

A benign tumour may undergo malignant changes. A malignant tumour of bone may be primary, or secondary as a result of a primary tumour elsewhere, when it is known as a *metastasis*.

Tumours may be classified according to the tissue from which they arise, e.g. chondroma from cartilage; osteosarcoma from bone.

Benign tumours are not generally a threat to life and may not require treatment unless they are interfering with the patient's ability to move, or are affecting the function of certain vital structures from pressure. A benign tumour will require treatment if it has a tendency to become malignant. Benign tumours may be treated by surgical removal.

Primary malignant tumours of bone are usually associated with pain. Treatment will depend on the type of tumour and its location. Osteosarcomas and Ewing's tumour tend to occur in the younger age-groups, whereas multiple myeloma tends to occur in the middle aged and elderly.

Secondary bone tumours (metastases) may develop following a primary tumour of the lung, prostate gland or the breast.

Methods of treatment include:
 i Chemotherapy.
 ii Radiotherapy.
 iii Hormone therapy.
 iv Surgical treatment.

Any one of the above may be used or a combination of any of them for maximum effectiveness and relief of pain.

RICKETS

This is a disease of childhood caused by deficiency of vitamin D. (Vitamin D deficiency in adults is termed osteomalacia.) It is a disease not commonly seen nowadays although it is being reported more among the Asian population. It is caused by inadequate intake of vitamin D in the diet or lack of sunlight. Vitamin D is required for the absorption of calcium and its utilization by the body. Deficiency therefore affects the normal development of bone with enlargement of the epiphysis. The bones become bent and pliable. Apart from the bony deformities, there is muscular weakness, anaemia, excessive sweating, diarrhoea and a susceptibility to infections such as bronchitis.

Treatment involves the administration of vitamin D and calcium. The orthopaedic treatment is designed to prevent deformity or correct it where it has occurred. Surgical treatment is sometimes required for the correction of deformity.

PRACTICE QUESTIONS

1 *What is meant by the following terms?*
   a Osteomyelitis
   b Blood-borne infection
   c Septic arthritis
   d Blood culture
   e Sequestrum
   f Involucrum
   g Brodie's abscess
   h Caseation
   i Mantoux test
   j Plaster bed
   k 'Cold' abscess
   l Ewing's tumour
   m Chondroma
   n Osteomalacia
   o 'Rickety rosary'
   Answer the following questions
   p Which organism most frequently causes osteomyelitis?
   q What does the term saucerization mean for the treatment of osteomyelitis?
   r What is a rigor?
   s List the possible side-effects of streptomycin.

 t Why are the sites for intramuscular injections of streptomycin alternated?
 u What is meant by Pott's paraplegia?
 v Describe what preventive measures may be taken in relation to rickets.
2 *Mark the following statements True or False:*
 a The removal of a necrosed piece of bone is a sequestrectomy.
 b Osteomyelitis is a blood-borne disease, commonly of childhood caused usually by the tubercle bacillus.
 c Infection of the bone may occur as a result of syphilis.
 d Excessive thickening of bones in adults is called acromegaly and occurs as a result of insufficient growth hormone.
 e An osteosarcoma is a benign tumour of bone.
 f Tuberculosis is a disease caused by the tubercle bacillus which may be of the human type or less commonly the bovine type.
 g 'Night sweats' are commonly associated with bone tumours.
 h Vitamin D is a fat-soluble vitamin required by the body for the absorption of calcium.
 i Deficiency of vitamin C as well as causing scurvy can affect the formation of bone.
 j Calcium is mobilized from the bones in a state of hyperparathyroidism.
3 *Discuss the following case history:*

Mrs Bradway is a 39-year-old married woman admitted to your ward with an acute exacerbation of rheumatoid arthritis. This is her second admission with this condition and the small joints of her hands are affected as well as the wrists. She has two children, a son aged 14 and a daughter aged 10. Her husband is a detective with the police force. Her parents are retired and live approximately 60 miles away.

Using a problem-solving approach describe the total management of Mrs Bradway while she is in hospital.

 Read the question again and then take time to think about it. It is appreciated that in the real situation you would have far more information than this to plan your nursing care (and more time!). However, from the information you are given and the knowledge you have already gained about nursing, attempt to answer the question. You may well find that the problems you have identified are not exactly the same as those found in the answer provided, or in the same order. That is of itself not important as we all think differently. The problems however should be related to Mrs Bradway, the goals realistic and the nursing measures should be designed to achieve those goals. Evaluation should be considered.

Orthopaedic Nursing

■ **Answers**

1 *a* An infection of the bone causing a disruption of the blood supply to the affected part. This together with toxins causes destruction of bone and the formation of pus.

  b An infection which develops in a part of the body as a result of being carried there by the blood.

  c Inflammation of the synovial membrane, also known as acute infective arthritis. In osteomyelitis it may develop as a result of spread from an adjacent bone. Septic arthritis can also develop as a result of wounds involving the joint, or following an infection elsewhere, e.g. scarlet fever. Other joint structures may become affected depending on the severity.

  d A specimen of blood which is obtained under aseptic conditions and transferred to a container containing a culture medium – this is later examined for micro-organisms.

  e A piece of dead bone which has become separated from the living tissue.

  f New bone which develops around necrosed bone. An involucrum surrounds a sequestrum.

  g A chronic bone abscess which is localized. It is treated by excision of the abscess and the wound is usually closed. Antibiotics are generally prescribed.

  h Changes that take place in the tissues in the presence of the tubercle bacilli giving rise to a 'cheesy mass'.

  i A test carried out to ascertain a person's susceptibility to tuberculosis.

  j A cast made of the whole of the patient's body so that he may be continuously nursed in the cast. An anterior shell is usually made so that periodically the patient is turned in the cast so that he may lie in the anterior shell. It may be ordered to secure immobilization in diseases affecting the spine.

  k A cold abscess is the term used to describe a type of tuberculous lesion.

  l A rapidly growing malignant tumour occurring in the young often before the age of 20. Treatment usually involves cytotoxic drugs and radiotherapy. The disease is almost always fatal.

  m A benign tumour arising from cartilage. Treatment is by excision if necessary.

  n A deficiency disease of adulthood due to inadequate amounts of vitamin D. In adults there is a tendency for bones to bend and to fracture.

  o A condition which may be seen in rickets as a result of enlargement of the costochondral junctions.

p *Staphylococcus aureus.*
q Radical clearance of an area in which there is much necrosed tissue and infection usually in chronic osteomyelitis. A prolonged course of antibiotics is usually prescribed to help eradicate the infection.
r A rigor is the body's attempt to deal with disturbances of temperature regulation. It is characterized by severe shivering and the patient's feeling cold as the body temperature rises. For management of the febrile patient see *Principles of Nursing* in this series.
s Skin rashes.
Damage to the VIIIth cranial nerve possibly leading to deafness.
Proteinuria.
t The drug is usually prescribed over a considerable period of time. It is therefore usual to alternate the sites to prevent the development of local irritations of the skin at the site of infection.
u A term used to describe paralysis of the lower limbs as a result of tuberculosis of the spine. It occurs as a result of the disease causing pressure on the spinal cord.
v Breast feeding.
Vitamin D supplements may be given in the form of drops if the baby is bottle fed.
Education regarding diet. Adequate exposure to sunlight.

2 a True
  b False
  c True
  d False
  e False
  f True
  g False
  h True
  i True
  j True

3 (Note: *The following is an example of one method which may be used to answer the question. Other methods may be used.*)

Rheumatoid arthritis is a non-suppurative inflammatory condition affecting the joints (most commonly the smaller joints) although the patient will feel ill in herself.

A problem-solving approach involves a systematic method of carrying out the nursing management of the patient. The nursing process is a tool which may be used for this purpose. The steps used for systematic care are assessment, planning, implementation and evaluation.

When Mrs Bradway arrives on the ward an assessment will be made of her condition and information gathered from all available sources. The conventional admission procedure will include the recording of vital signs and a ward test of a specimen of urine. When she is comfortably positioned in bed a nursing history can then be obtained, preferably in the form of a conversation with the minimum of distraction.

Planning will then proceed as problems are identified. The goal is then stated for each problem as a measure against which the evaluation of the nursing care can be made. Mrs Bradway's problems may include the following:

	Problem	Goal
1 (A)	Pain in the hands and wrists.	Alleviate the pain.
2 (A)	Inability to maintain personal hygiene.	Maintain personal hygiene.
3 (A)	Difficulty with eating and drinking.	Maintain fluid balance and nutritional state of patient.
4 (A)	Feeling weak and tired.	Reduce feeling of weakness and tiredness.
5 (A)	Loss of independence.	Gradual restoration of independence.
6 (A)	Anxious regarding care of children.	Less anxious about family.
7 (P)	Pressure sore formation, muscle wasting and joint contractures.	Skin will remain intact.

Key — (A) actual (P) potential.

This stage can then be followed by formulating the nursing instructions for implementation.

1 Pain
Maintain splintage as advised by the surgeon. Physiotherapist attending twice daily and carrying out passive movements. Analgesia and anti-inflammatory drugs administered as prescribed.
Handle splinted limbs gently.
Firm base to bed, correct use of pillows and maintenance of posture.
Light bed clothes. One blanket (loose).
Diversional therapy
   i Talking to patient
   ii Radio/television
   iii Newspapers/books
Ask occupational therapist to visit patient.
These measures are then evaluated at regular intervals.

2 Personal hygiene
Blanket bath patient/daily.
Freshening wash in the evening.

Clean teeth morning and evening.
Mouthwashes – after meals.
Nails – keep short, clean and manicured.
Wash hair – once weekly.
Use patient's own talcum powder and deodorants.

On evaluation further measures may be required if the patient is pyrexial and perspiring.

3 Eating and drinking
Feed patient at mealtimes.
Husband bringing in cold chicken salad for Tuesday/Friday evenings.
Cup of tea to be taken with meals.
Milk drink to be given at 9 a.m., 10 a.m., 2 p.m., 5 p.m.
Cup of Horlicks at 9 p.m. before retiring.
Maintain fluid balance chart.

Following removal of splintage the plan will be modified so that the patient can feed herself if the meat is cut up for her, and lightweight cups used for drinking. Water jug can be half filled so that she can pour her own drinks. The plan may alter again when she is eating at the table.

4 Weak and tired
2 units of blood given as ordered by the doctor.
One-hourly observations of vital signs while transfusion is in progress.
One hour rest periods – (10–11 a.m.) (2–3 p.m.)
Give bed time drink at 9 p.m.
Give sedation as prescribed.
Two head pillows removed for the night.
Turn lights down at 10 p.m.
Not to be woken until 8 a.m.

As the patient responds the plan may be modified slightly.

5 Independence
Ask doctor to explain to the patient the reason for her discomfort.
Explain why splintage is necessary and the importance of rest.
Inform her that as the acute period subsides she will begin to feel well again, and be able to do things for herself.
Give bedpans with minimum of fuss.
Use female urinal to try and reduce feeling of being a burden.

Response to nursing measures are evaluated. It may be necessary to seek the doctor's permission for the patient to get up to use a commode – this may lead to a feeling of greater independence.

6 *Care of children*
Discuss home situation with patient and husband.
Ask husband to keep wife informed.
Children to come and see mother in the evenings – 6 p.m. as
hospital visiting is late for the younger child.

On evaluation – adaptation of visiting times to accommodate the younger child resolved much of the anxiety. Immediate resolution was achieved by the husband taking two days leave giving the grandparents time to organize themselves to come and stay with the family.

7 *Pressure sore formation, muscle wasting/joint contractures*
Place sheepskin along whole length of the bed.
Change patient's position 2-hourly.
Lift and move patient gently, replace pillows correctly for support and maintenance of position.
Ensure feet are supported and kept in neutral position.
Ask physiotherapist to assess the patient.
Note the patient's skin and heels on each turn.
Always leave sheepskin flat and smooth.

The time taken to achieve the goals will vary and other problems may arise during the course of time. Preparation for discharge home will be carried out in the same way. The medical social worker may have to be involved. The patient is involved throughout with the planning of her care.

7 Conditions affecting children

In this chapter some of the conditions which affect children are described. Spina bifida is included because developing deformities may require orthopaedic surgery.
1. Congenital abnormalities:
   a Congenital dislocation of the hip (CDH).
   b Congenital talipes equinovarus.
   c Spina bifida.
2 The management of a child with Perthes' disease.
3 Scoliosis and an outline of the management.
(Osteomyelitis is discussed in Chapter 6)

■ CONGENITAL ABNORMALITIES

Children born with orthopaedic abnormalities are likely to undergo treatment and certainly supervision by the orthopaedic surgeon for many years. Conditions such as congenital dislocation of the hip/s and talipes are generally diagnosed nowadays at the time of birth or within a few weeks. This is obviously advantageous as it means that treatment can begin almost immediately, within hours of the birth in some instances. It usually means for the parents that they have to come to terms with some degree of physical defect. It is not usual at this time to consider how the child will feel when he/she has to undergo surgery perhaps for the second, third or even more times by the time he/she is 10 years old. For much of that time the child may not be undergoing any kind of treatment other than attending the outpatient department for regular check-ups. Generally the child adapts well to the situation probably because he/she knows nothing different. It isn't perhaps until a brother or a sister comes along who is born without a congenital defect that the older infant will wonder why he has to wear splints in bed and the baby does not.

When a baby or child is admitted into hospital it is usually the nurse who greets the mother and child and carries out the admission procedure and nursing interview. Special consideration is given to babies, infants and children and relevant information obtained including the feeding regime, daily naps, sleeping pattern, use of dummies, bed times, favourite drinks, toys and so on. The baby may 'suck' a small blanket or cloth when he goes to sleep, in which case great care must be taken to ensure that it is not lost – or finds its way to the hospital laundry! If such things seem unimportant – they are not. If the mother has brought the article into hospital, it is a source of comfort for the child and provides a link between home and hospital which must be maintained. If the mother can stay with the child then this should be encouraged.

Much has been written in recent years about the possible effects of hospitalization on the child and the nurse should be aware of them. It is not expected that nurses should know exactly how the parents feel because this is not always possible; it is possible, however, to listen, to talk, to show an interest and build up a meaningful relationship with both the child and the parents. Involvement of the parents is of particular importance because for some children much of the treatment may be done as an outpatient, so that the child will be cared for at home.

Finally, mention is made about the upheaval that a hospitalization causes for the family and the arrangements and adjustments that have to be made. It is perhaps a mistake to assume that because children with orthopaedic congenital abnormalities often undergo intermittent periods of hospitalization over a number of years that parents get used to it. It is more likely that each admission causes the same amount of disruption for the family, it may be easier in the sense that they have some idea of what to expect, but each admission is different. So rather than 'get used to it' it is more than likely that each time they have to be resourceful enough to cope with it differently. The degree and kind of support they will require each time will vary, as will the support they have to give to the child.

■ Congenital dislocation of the hip (CDH)

This condition, as the term suggests, means that the child (more commonly girls) is born with complete or partial dislocation of the hip joint, i.e. the femoral head is displaced from the acetabulum. One or both hips may be affected. It is thought that perhaps the disorder develops late in intra-uterine life due to factors which cause the acetabulum to be shallower than normal and insufficiently developed to accommodate the femoral head, and the laxity of soft tissue structures surrounding the joint. The babies are often a breech presentation.

Changes will take place in the femoral head, acetabulum, and the surrounding soft tissues if the condition continues undiagnosed.

□ *Diagnosis*

It is obviously preferable for the condition to be diagnosed as early as possible so that treatment may be commenced. If there is a history of congenital dislocation of hip in the family then the baby will be particularly closely examined at birth. *All* newborn babies are carefully examined by the paediatrician and if there are signs of CDH the opinion of the orthopaedic surgeon is sought. Signs which may be present include an abnormally wide perineum and legs which cannot be fully abducted. The surgeon will carry out various manipulative tests on the hip joint to establish the presence of a 'click', as the head of femur slips over the acetabular rim (Ortolani's sign). The joints of a young baby are at all times handled very carefully and gently. Radiological examination will confirm the diagnosis and indicate the extent of displacement. Occasionally a child will be brought for an opinion after walking has commenced, when it has been noticed that one leg appears to be better developed than the other or that one leg appears to be longer. A limp may also be present. There is usually limitation of movement, a prominent lordosis and greater trochanter, and if both sides are affected the limbs may appear short in relation to the size of the body. Trendelenburg's sign may be present when the pelvis drops to the unaffected side as the patient stands on the affected limb.

□ *Treatment*

Treatment is commenced as early as possible so that the hip joint may continue to develop normally. If the condition is detected at birth reduction of the dislocation is relatively simple. Immobilization can then be maintained by means of a splint, e.g. Barlow splint, or van Rosen splint (Fig. 14) for a period of approximately three months. The advantage of this kind of splint is that the baby can be cared for at home with regular visits to the outpatient department. It is important that the mother understands the need for the splintage and her co-operation in the management of the child is sought.

It may be necessary for reduction to be carried out gradually over a period of time by means of traction and/or an abduction frame. Different types of traction may be used for this purpose. Some restrict the child considerably whereas in comparison others are unrestricted while still retaining the traction force. During this time the child's mother is allowed to visit and be with the child as much as she can. Consideration should be given to the mother and the nurse should be sensitive to the fact that the mother cannot do what she very often would instinctively do for the child, such as picking her up and cuddling her. Following reduction, some form of immobilization may be ordered either in the form of a splint or a plaster cast. A frog plaster may be applied extending from the nipple line to the ankle, maintaining the hips in abduction and external rotation (Fig. 15).

Care of the plaster is important and in particular to prevent its soiling by urine and faeces. Wooden seats and frames have been designed to facilitate the management of a child in frog plasters. Usually the child can be allowed

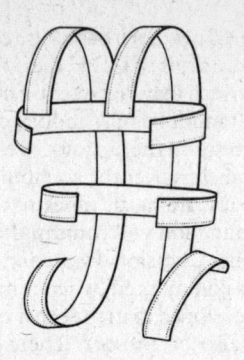

Fig. 14 van Rosen splint

to do what she can within the limitations imposed by the plaster. The cast may be retained for up to nine months or more, until the joint is considered to be stable. Sometimes the plaster may be removed and the child allowed to kick free in bed, at other times successive plasters may be applied before final removal to reduce gradually the positions of abduction and external rotation and to then allow the child freedom in bed.

Operative treatment may be required particularly with the older child where manipulative reduction is difficult. The type of surgery performed depends on changes present in the hip. Surgery is followed by a period of immobilization on similar lines to that already described.

■ **Talipes equinovarus** (club foot) (Fig. 16)

In this condition the child is born with deformity of the foot or feet commonly called club foot/feet. The deformity consists of adduction of the forefoot, inversion of the foot, plantar flexion and occasionally rotation of the tibia.

When the condition is bilateral, one foot is usually more severely deformed than the other. The sooner this deformity is detected and treated the better.

□ *Treatment*
Correction of the deformity is the aim of treatment, and in babies detected at birth this is effected by manipulation and thereafter the foot/feet held in the overcorrected position by some form of splintage e.g. adhesive strapping, Denis Browne splints, Bell-Grice splints or plaster of Paris fixation.

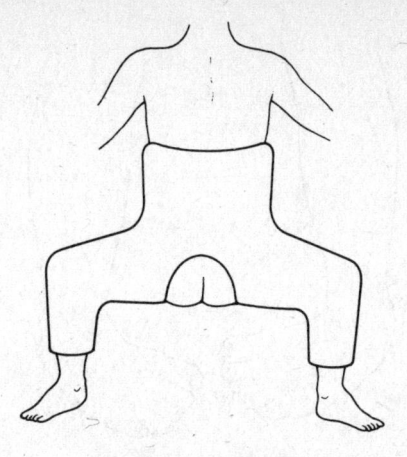

Fig. 15 Frog plaster

Initially the feet are re-manipulated and fixation re-applied frequently, e.g. at weekly intervals. The baby is treated as an outpatient although the first manipulation is probably done while the mother and baby are still in the maternity wing of the hospital. The advantage of this method of conservative treatment is that the mother can take the baby home with her. The first year or so will involve frequent visits to the outpatient department and at each time circulation to the toes is checked before the baby is allowed to leave the clinic. The co-operation of the mother is required and the importance of maintaining the splintage throughout is explained to her at the outset. It may be that below-knee plaster of Paris will be maintained until the child is walking. The mother and baby miss out on what are usually considered to be enjoyable bath times during this period but if plaster of Paris is used the mother may later be allowed to soak the plasters off in the bath the night before attending clinic – this ritual is then very precious and makes up for those missed bath times. The fact that the baby has below-knee plasters on appears not to interfere with normal motor development and when the baby walks the plasters are usually discarded and the first pair of shoes is bought in the usual way.

☐ *Management*
Alterations may be made to the shoes as prescribed by the surgeon so that the position achieved by previous treatment can be maintained. Denis Browne splints may be worn during the night. This may continue for a

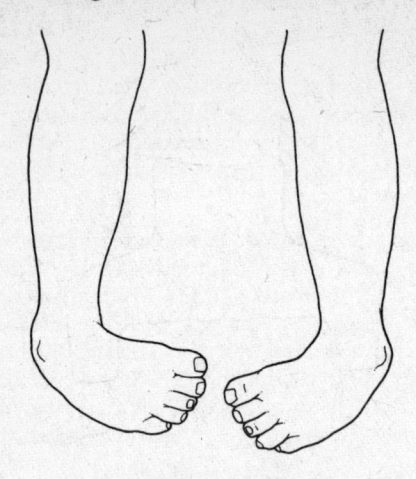

Fig. 16 Talipes equinovarus

number of years, each new pair of shoes being altered until such time as the surgeon states otherwise. It may be at some time during the course of treatment that elongation of the tendon achilles (ETA) will be required. This is a procedure which involves staying in hospital overnight and the tenotomy is followed by a period of approximately six weeks in plaster.

□ *Surgery*
Supervision by the orthopaedic surgeon is continued throughout the growing life of the child and surgery may be advised at any time during the course of these years so that the deformity is controlled. When the child is five years or over it may be necessary for bone surgery to be carried out, such as the (Dilwyn Evans) procedure where a wedge resection of the cuboid and calcaneum is made accompanied by surgery on the soft tissue structures. The limb is then placed in plaster of Paris. Sutures are removed under anaesthetic in approximately 14 days followed by re-application of plaster. Plaster fixation is retained for approximately four months. The child is usually allowed to weight-bear (and a walking plaster applied) on the surgeon's instructions, approximately 8 weeks following surgery. Following final removal of plaster a crêpe bandage or a Tubigrip bandage/sock is worn for a few days to prevent the development of oedema.

In cases where persistent deformity recurs stabilization of the foot may be required by carrying out arthrodeses of the joints of the foot (triple arthrodesis).

■ Spina bifida

Spina bifida is a congenital abnormality affecting the spine. Due to defective development of the spinal column its contents may protrude through a gap. There are varying degrees of spina bifida and the deformities present will depend on the extent to which the spinal cord is involved.

□ *Spina bifida occulta*

The laminae on the posterior aspect of the vertebrae fail to fuse or do not develop properly – there may be a pad of horny skin with a tuft of hairs overlying the defect. The spinal cord or its coverings are not involved and usually no treatment is required. If the bony defect is more extensive the membrane of the spinal cord may protrude through the bony defect, and although the spinal cord itself does not protrude the sac usually contains cerebrospinal fluid. Treatment consists of early surgical management of the sac and the prognosis is generally satisfactory. This defect is known as a meningocele.

□ *A meningomyelocele*

This defect consists of the protrusion containing the spinal cord and nerve tissue. These are more common in the lumbar-sacral region, the child may be paralysed from the waist down with bladder and bowel involvement. Some may also develop hydrocephalus. Surgery is aimed at closing the defect, covering exposed nerve tissue, minimizing paralysis and preventing infection. Babies are usually nursed in incubators at this time so that body temperature can be maintained. Hydrocephalus may be treated by the insertion of a valve for shunting the cerebrospinal fluid via the jugular vein into the venous system, e.g. Spitz-Holter valve. As soon as the mother feels well enough she is encouraged to visit the baby and as soon as possible will be able to feed, bath and change him. Needless to say untiring support must be given to the parents not only at this time but continuously in different ways for many years to come.

Management of the bladder and bowels will require attention, the aim being to achieve continence. Whatever treatment is found to be necessary every effort should be made to enhance the physical and mental development of the child.

■ Perthes' disease

This is an abnormality of the hip joint. It is not congenital and commonly occurs about the age of 6 or 7 years. It occurs more often in boys. Both hips may be affected. It is a non-inflammatory disease affecting the epiphysis and the supply of blood to the femoral head. (The lesion can occur at any epiphyseal site but when it affects the upper femoral epiphysis it is called Perthes' disease.)

The child may be seen to be limping but is uncomplaining. The child may complain of an ache or even pain which may be referred to the knee. On examination abduction and rotation movements are limited. There may also be flexion contracture of the hip joint present. The disease heals spontaneously in about two to three years.

□ *Treatment*

The aim of treatment is to rest the joint until the femoral head appears to be healing, regular radiological examination of the joint is ordered so that the stages of change which the head of femur undergoes can be monitored. The child is nursed in bed either with or without traction. The exact treatment depends on the surgeon but the aim is to achieve rest of the affected part. The length of time spent in bed/on traction varies also, and when the child is up, non-weight-bearing is achieved by the use of a patten-end caliper, hip sling or the Birmingham splint. Time spent in hospital usually extends over a number of weeks so that education is continued in hospital. Sometimes operative treatment may be carried out. The above-mentioned splints may be used following surgery as a means of obtaining mobilization without bearing weight. The physiotherapist is involved at all stages of the treatment.

■ Scoliosis (Fig. 17)

This is a lateral curvature of the spine with rotation.

The scoliosis may be secondary to some other condition in which case treatment is aimed at the cause. It may be congenital or it may be caused by persistently adopting a bad posture. It may be due to factors affecting the soft tissues in the region of the spine or it may be idiopathic. (In the majority of cases there is no known cause.)

Apart from the obvious deformity the patient may complain of backache and later pain. If the deformity is as a result of poor posture, exercises and re-education is required. The physiotherapist will instruct the patient regarding special exercises.

□ *Treatment*

The treatment for structural scoliosis depends on the age of the child and the severity of the condition. Management may be conservative or surgical or a combination of both. Treatment may extend over a period of years. Different forms of splintage may be used in an attempt to correct the

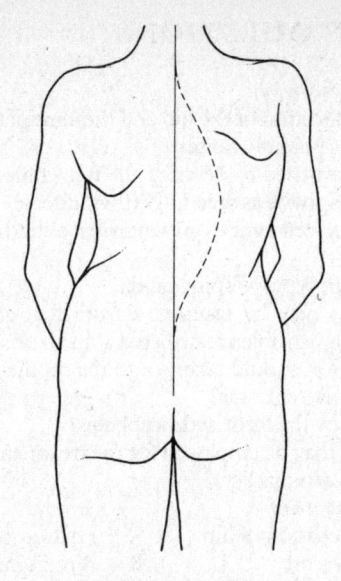

Fig. 17 Scoliosis

deformity or prevent the progress of the deformity until such time as an operative procedure may be performed.

A *Milwaukee brace* which extends from the pelvis to the chin helps to maintain the spine in a position of extension.

A *turnbuckle plaster jacket* may be used for gradual correction of the deformity. Following correction a spinal fusion may then be performed through a window cut in the plaster.

Correction can also be achieved by means of *halo-pelvic traction*. This comprises a halo attached to the skull by means of pins and a hoop attached to the pelvis by means of pins also. Extension bars are then attached to the halo above and the pelvic hoop below. Gradual correction is achieved by distraction; because of possible traction on the spinal cord, neurological observations are made. When maximum correction has been achieved a spinal fusion may be performed. The halo-pelvic device is maintained until the fusion is united.

Internal correction of the deformity and its maintenance may be achieved by the insertion of Harrington rods. The surgery is a major procedure and the patient is prepared accordingly. The postoperative management may involve immobilization on a plaster bed for up to three months postoperatively and a further three months in a plaster jacket.

PRACTICE QUESTIONS

1 *Briefly explain the following:*
   a Congenital dislocation of the hip and the aims of treatment.
   b Scoliosis and its possible causes.
   c What is the term used to describe the non-inflammatory condition affecting the epiphysis as seen in Perthes' disease?
   d What may be the deformities present when a child is born with talipes equinovarus?
   e List the different types of spina bifida.
   f What measures may be taken to ensure that as many congenital abnormalities as possible are detected at birth or soon afterwards?
   g What information should be given to the mother before she takes a child in a frog plaster home?
   h What is meant by the term hydrocephalus?
   i What methods may be employed for the treatment of scoliosis?
   j A turnbuckle plaster jacket.

2 *Match the following items:*
   a Congenital dislocation of hip   A   Hydrocephalus.
   b Talipes equinovarus.   B   Birmingham splint.
   c Perthes' disease.   C   Frog plasters.
   d Scoliosis   D   Elongation of tendon achilles.
   e Spina bifida   E   Milwaukee brace.

3 *Complete the following sentences:*
   a Lateral curvature of the spine is termed _____.
   b 'Mushrooming' of the femoral head occurs in _____.
   c Harrington rods may be used to correct the deformity of _____.
   d Hydrocephalus may be treated by the insertion of a shunting valve called _____.
   e A sac on the surface of the baby's back (spina bifida) containing CSF and no nerve tissue is called a _____.
   f A defect which is present at birth is said to be _____.
   g A defect for which there appears to be no known cause is called _____.
   h Manipulation of the hip joint with the presence of a 'click' as the head of femur slips over the acetabulum is termed _____ sign.
   i A Barlow or van Rosen splint is used for the treatment of _____.
   j Triple arthrodesis may be performed as treatment for the older child with _____.

4 *Mark the following questions True or False:*
   a Forcible manipulation of congenital hip dislocation may give rise to Perthes' disease.

b Congenital talipes equinovarus is commoner in girls than boys.
c The cause of congenital talipes equinovarus is not known.
d Congenital dislocation of the hip is commoner in girls than boys.
e During the manipulation of a club foot the knee should be protected by an assistant.
f Perthes' disease is caused by inflammation of the hip joint.
g Some types of congenital talipes equinovarus are severe and difficult to treat, relapse of the condition being common.
h A Spitz-Holter valve drains CSF via the jugular vein into the inferior vena cava.
i Scoliosis, kyphosis and lordosis are all conditions of the spine.
j Perthes' disease is a congenital disease.

■ Answers

1 *a* The child is born with partial or complete displacement of the femoral head from the acetabulum. Both hips may be affected. The aim of treatment includes reduction of the displacement and its maintenance so that normal development of the joint can continue.
  b Lateral curvature of the spine. The curves include a *primary* curve which develops from the possible cause and the *secondary* curves are those that compensate the primary curve. Scoliosis may develop from an abnormality of the spine itself or following a disease process affecting the spine, e.g. osteoarthritis, tuberculosis, tumours. If the spine does not develop properly the scoliosis may be congenital. It may occur following diseases affecting muscles, as a result of paralysis such as poliomyelitis, or it may be idiopathic.
  c Osteochondritis.
  d Plantar flexion, inversion of the foot, adduction of the forefoot and possibly rotation of the tibia medially.
  e Spina bifida occulta; meningocele; meningomyelocele; anterior spina bifida; myelocele.
  f Babies born in the United Kingdom undergo a complete physical examination known as 'examination of the newborn'. Obvious deformities at birth are noted and referred appropriately, others may be observed on examination by the paediatrician. Clinics are also available for the mother to attend with the baby at regular intervals and periodically the baby will be examined by a doctor, so that any defects not detected at birth may be noted soon afterwards. Midwives and health visitors also visit the home following discharge so that the mother may be kept informed of clinic attendances and so on.
  g The plaster would be dried in hospital prior to discharge home. The

importance of avoiding soiling of the plaster is impressed on the mother, as this will cause softening and lead to possible soreness of the skin and the loss of the effectiveness of the splint. If the child is of an age to control bowel and bladder she will be advised regarding wooden perches and stools that may be used for the purposes of using the 'potty'. In a young child who is not trained, the genital region of the plaster may be protected by waterproof adhesive tape to avoid contamination, and the mother is advised not to let the nappies get too wet, that is, to change them frequently.

  h Hydrocephalus is a term used to describe enlargement of the head due to an accumulation of cerebrospinal fluid.
  i Conservative method, e.g. plaster casts, Milwaukee brace.
Operative treatment, insertion of Harrington rods, spinal fusion.
Combination of both.
  j A plaster cast encasing the trunk which may include the head and a shoulder. The plaster is split transversely and a turnbuckle is applied to the two halves of the cast. Correction is achieved gradually by manipulation of the turnbuckle causing the two halves of the plaster to open out at a level which is approximated to the deformity.

2 *a* C
  b D
  c B
  d E
  e A.

3 *a* Scoliosis
  b Perthes' disease
  c Scoliosis
  d Spitz-Holter
  e Meningocele
  f Congenital
  g Idiopathic
  h Ortolani's
  i Congenital dislocation of the hip
  j Congenital talipes equinovarus.

4 *a* True
  b False
  c True
  d True
  e True
  f False
  g True

h False
i True
j False.

Advice for examination preparation

Start your preparation well in advance of the examination. Make a realistic plan of action that you will be able to achieve.
1. Decide how many hours each day you can set aside for study/revision. 2 hours daily × 5 = 10 hours weekly.
2. Make a timetable and slot in all the subjects to be studied. The length of time you allocate depends on the level of difficulty.
3. Study in the same place each day. Sit at a desk or table and have the materials you need at hand – paper, pencils, crayons, textbooks, lecture notes and a rubber. Write in pencil so that mistakes or unwanted notes can be erased (paper is expensive).
4. You must work at concentrating on your task; don't allow yourself to think of anything else so that you waste time.
5. If you are tired or upset, relax before attempting to settle.
6. Work at each of the goals you have set yourself as widely as you can.
7. Reward yourself when a goal is achieved so that you associate pleasure with studying.
8. Success is not a matter of luck but of good planning and self-discipline.
9. Learning is an active process so:
   - Study using a logical approach. Sequence the material and go from easy to more difficult concepts.
   - Don't try to learn chunks of material; skim the passage and try to understand. Underline key words or sentences. Use a dictionary.
   - Consciously recall and reinforce your memory. Commit your thoughts to paper.
   - Use mnemonics as a memory aid.
   - Ask yourself questions, apply the material, compare with management of actual patients you have nursed. Have discussions with friends/tutors.
   - Ask your tutors for help if you do not understand the relevance of a topic.
   - Learn to draw and label line-drawings correctly.
   - Test yourself using past examination questions.
   - Get a relative or friend to ask you questions.
10. Cultivate a fast reading style. Use several textbooks with your notes. Make your own notes when you have analysed the meaning of a

passage. Begin to read with a question in mind and ask yourself questions when you have read a paragraph/chapter. Read quickly then re-read.
11 What you want to achieve is efficiency of study with economy of effort.

■ EXAMINATION TECHNIQUE

1 Listen to any instructions and follow them carefully. Be prepared with pens, pencils, a rubber and ruler.
2 Read the instructions on the examination paper and comply with them, i.e. start a question on a fresh page, number your questions carefully, write legibly. Note how many questions are to be attempted, how much time is allowed, etc.
3 Essay questions test:
   o Knowledge
   o Comprehension
   o Application
   o Communication
   o Synthesis.
4 Read all the questions carefully on both sides of the paper, identify all parts of each question before starting to answer.
   o Don't be concerned that others have started to write.
   o Select the questions you feel most able to answer.
   o Tick your selection in order of sequence.
   o Analyse the setting of the question. Is the scene in hospital or the community? What is the importance of age, sex, marital/social status, environment, psychological well-being, needs of the patient in the examiner's mind. Underline these points and develop them.
   o Note the essential points that have to be made in your answer in the margin of the paper.
   o Pay attention to the weighting of each part of the question; these should help you plan the time to be spent on each part.
   o Ten minutes spent in planning is the most effective way of using the examination time.
   o When you start to write:
   Answer the parts in order of a, b, c, d.
   Write legibly, be logical (first things first).
   Concentrate on the main parts, don't waffle and repeat yourself.
   If a diagram is asked for, make a clear line drawing and label it clearly.
   Leave time at the end for reading your answers.

108 Orthopaedic Nursing

Remember that a good essay has an introduction, a development and a conclusion, and should be clear and concise. Remember also that each sentence requires a verb.

Further reading

BEDBROOK, G. (1981). *The Care and Management of the Spinal Cord*. Springer-Verlag, New York.
BROMLEY, I. (1980). *Tetraplegia and Paraplegia*, 2nd edition. Churchill Livingstone, Edinburgh.
BRUNNER, L. S. and SUDDATH, D. S. (1987). *The Lippincott Manual of Medical-Surgical Nursing*, Volume 3. Harper and Row, London.
FARRELL, J. (1986). *Illustrated Guide to Orthopaedic Nursing*, 3rd edition. Harper and Row, London.
FOOTNER, A. (1987). *Orthopaedic Nursing*. Baillière Tindall, London.
POWELL, M. (ed.) (1986). *Orthopaedic Nursing and Rehabilitation*, 9th edition. Churchill Livingstone, Edinburgh.

The following two references are specific to arthroplasty:
AUGUST, A. C., ALDAM, C. H. and PYNSENT, P. B. (1986). The McKee-Farrar hip arthroplasty – a long-term study. *Journal of Bone and Joint Surgery* (Br), **68B**, 520–7.
RYD, L. (1986). Micromotion in knee arthroplasty. *Acta Orthopedica Scandinavica* (Supp 220), **57**.

Index

admission, emergency, 35
  of patients, 1
  psychological factors of, 3–4
annulus fibrosus, 41, 42
arthroplasty, of hip, 69, 73–5
Austin Moore prosthesis, 25, 71

balanced traction, 8
  use in fractured femur, 25, 31
Barlow splint, 95
Bell Grice splints, 96
bladder care, in paraplegia, 50
bone, classification, 20–21
  healing of, 21–2
  infection of (osteomyelitis), 78–81
  structure of, 19–21
  tuberculosis of, 81–5
  tumours of, 85
bowel care, 5, 12, 29
  in paraplegia, 51
Braun splint, 33
Bryant's traction, 32

callus, 21, 22
cancellous bone, 19
cast brace, 21–2
clavicle, fracture of, 24
Colles' fracture, 24
communication, with patients and/or relatives, 3–4, 30, 66–7, 80, 84
  relating to cast care, 15–16
  relating to paraplegia, 52–4
compact bone, 19
compound fractures, 35
congenital abnormalities in children, 93–101
  CDH, 94–6
  spina bifida, 99
  talipes equinovarus, 96–9

congenital dislocation of hip (CDH), 94–6
crepitus, 22, 38(r)

Denham's pin, 10
Denis Browne splints, 96, 97
'dinner fork' deformity, 24
drug, administration, 6
  therapy, in bone tuberculosis, 82
    in osteomyelitis, 80
    in rheumatoid arthritis, 64
drying of splintage materials:
  plaster of Paris, 13–14
  Scotch/Delta Lite casts, 15

elimination, 5, 28–9, 66, 80, 84
elongation of tendon achilles (ETA), 98
ethambutol, 82

fat embolism, 39(c)
femur fractures, of neck, 25
  of shaft, 31–2
  in small children, 32
figure-of-eight bandage, 24
fixed traction, 8, 31
fractures, 19–36
  classification, 22–3
  of lower limbs, 25, 31–4
  management of, 34–6
  of pelvis, 34
  repair of, 21
  of upper limbs, 24–5
frog plaster, 95, 97

gallows traction *see* Bryant's traction

halo-pelvic traction, 101
Hamilton Russell traction, 8, 10, 25, 29

Harrington rods, 101
Haversian system, 19, 21
health education, for bone
 tuberculosis, 84–5
human tetanus immunoglobulins, 35
humerus, fractures of, 24
Humotet, 35
hydrocephalus, 99
hygiene, 4, 27, 49, 64, 79, 83

isoniazid, 82

joints, affected in osteoarthritis, 67
 affected in rheumatoid arthritis,
  63
 replacement of *see* arthroplasty
 structure and function, 59–60
 synovial, 60

Kirschner wire, 10
knee joint, 60–61
Kuntscher intramedullary nail, 31

laminectomy, 43
'log rolling', 43, 44
low back pain, 42, *see* prolapsed
 intervertebral disc

McKee Farrar hip replacement, 70
meningomyelocele, 99
meniscectomy, 60–62
metastasis, 85
micturition, 5, 28
 in paraplegia, 50–51
Milwaukee brace, 101
mobilization/mobility of patients, 6,
 29, 79, 83
 after hip replacement, 71, 74–5
 in paraplegia, 51–2
 in rheumatoid arthritis, 65
muscles, structure, 59

Norton scale, 4, 83
Norwich cementless hip replacement,
 73–5
nucleus pulposus, 41, 42

nursing management:
 bone tuberculosis, 83–4
 childhood conditions, 93–101
 elderly patients, 26–30
 hip arthroplasty, 70–73
 infants, 33
 laminectomy, 43–4
 meniscectomy, 62
 osteoarthritis, 69–73
 osteomyelitis, 79–81
 paraplegia, 46–54
 plaster casts, 13–14
 rheumatoid arthritis, 64–7, 87(3),
  89(3)–92
 Scotch/Delta Lite casts, 15
 traction, 10–12
nutrition, 4–5, 27, 49, 65–6, 79, 83

occupational therapy, 30
 in paraplegia, 49, 52
orthopaedic, nursing, principles of,
 1–7
 ward, 1–2
Ortolani's sign, 95
osteoarthritis, 67–73
 surgery for, 68
  management after, 69–73
 treatment, 68
osteoblasts, 19
osteoclasts, 20
osteomyelitis, 78–81
osteophytes, 67
osteotomy, 68, 69

paraplegia, 45
 chest care in, 49
 nursing management, 46–54
 psychological management, 52–4
pelvis, fracture of, 34
periosteum, 19, 21
Perthes' disease, 99–100
physiotherapy, 30
 for low backache, 43
 for meniscectomy, 62
 for osteoarthritis, 68, 72–3, 74–5
 for paraplegia, 49, 51–2

for rheumatoid arthritis, 65
plaster of Paris, drying of, 13–14
  use for immobilization, 13
plaster casts/splints, 13–14
positioning of patient with
    paraplegia, 47–8
Pott's fracture, 33
pressure sores, in paraplegia, 50
prolapsed intervertebral disc
    (lumbar), 42–4
  conservative treatment, 43
  laminectomy for, 43–4

rehabilitation, 7
  of the paraplegic/tetraplegic, 52
rest/sleep, 30, 66, 84
rheumatoid arthritis, 62–7
  medical treatment, 64
  nursing management, 64–7
rickets, 86
Robert Jones' bandage, 62

scoliosis, 100–101, 103(1b)
shock (after fracture), 35
skeletal traction, 10
  for fracture of tibia and fibula, 33
  nursing observations, 11
skeleton, functions of, 21
skin care, 4, 27, 49, 64–5, 79, 83
skin traction, 9
  nursing observations, 10
sliding traction *see* balanced traction
spina bifida, 99
spine, anatomy of, 41
  curvature of, 100–101
  injury to, 45–6

Spitz-Holter valve, 99
splints, 12–13
  care, when wearing, 65
  for CDH, 95, 96
  for talipes equinovarus, 96
Steinmann's pin, 10
streptomycin, 82

talipes equinovarus, 96–9
  splintage for, 97
  surgery for, 98
Thomas' bed splint, 8, 9, 13, 31, 33
Thompson prosthesis, 25
tibia and fibula, fracture, 33
tincture of benzoin, use with skin
    traction, 9
traction, types, 8–9, 10
  halo-pelvic, 101
  methods of application, 9–10
  nursing management, 10–12
Trendelenburg's sign, 95
tuberculosis of bone, 81–5
  drug therapy for, 82
  health education for, 84
tumours of bone, 85
turnbuckle plaster jacket, 101

urine, 5, 28

van Rosen splint, 95, 96
vertebrae, 41, 42
Volkmann's ischaemic contracture,
    24, 38(i)

Waterlow scale, 4, 83

FOR THE BEST IN PAPERBACKS, LOOK FOR THE 🐧

In every corner of the world, on every subject under the sun, Penguin represents quality and variety – the very best in publishing today.

For complete information about books available from Penguin – including Pelicans, Puffins, Peregrines and Penguin Classics – and how to order them, write to us at the appropriate address below. Please note that for copyright reasons the selection of books varies from country to country.

In the United Kingdom: Please write to *Dept E.P., Penguin Books Ltd, Harmondsworth, Middlesex, UB7 0DA*

If you have any difficulty in obtaining a title, please send your order with the correct money, plus ten per cent for postage and packaging, to *PO Box No 11, West Drayton, Middlesex*

In the United States: Please write to *Dept BA, Penguin, 299 Murray Hill Parkway, East Rutherford, New Jersey 07073*

In Canada: Please write to *Penguin Books Canada Ltd, 2801 John Street, Markham, Ontario L3R 1B4*

In Australia: Please write to the *Marketing Department, Penguin Books Australia Ltd, P.O. Box 257, Ringwood, Victoria 3134*

In New Zealand: Please write to the *Marketing Department, Penguin Books (NZ) Ltd, Private Bag, Takapuna, Auckland 9*

In India: Please write to *Penguin Overseas Ltd, 706 Eros Apartments, 56 Nehru Place, New Delhi, 110019*

In Holland: Please write to *Penguin Books Nederland B.V., Postbus 195, NL–1380AD Weesp, Netherlands*

In Germany: Please write to *Penguin Books Ltd, Friedrichstrasse 10–12, D–6000 Frankfurt Main 1, Federal Republic of Germany*

In Spain: Please write to *Longman Penguin España, Calle San Nicolas 15, E–28013 Madrid, Spain*

In France: Please write to *Penguin Books Ltd, 39 Rue de Montmorency, F-75003, Paris, France*

In Japan: Please write to *Longman Penguin Japan Co Ltd, Yamaguchi Building, 2–12–9 Kanda Jimbocho, Chiyoda-Ku, Tokyo 101, Japan*

FOR THE BEST IN PAPERBACKS, LOOK FOR THE 🐧

PENGUIN HEALTH

Audrey Eyton's F-Plus Audrey Eyton

'Your short cut to the most sensational diet of the century' – *Daily Express*

Baby and Child Penelope Leach

A beautifully illustrated and comprehensive handbook on the first five years of life. 'It stands head and shoulders above anything else available at the moment' – Mary Kenny in the *Spectator*

Woman's Experience of Sex Sheila Kitzinger

Fully illustrated with photographs and line drawings, this book explores the riches of women's sexuality at every stage of life. 'A book which any mother could confidently pass on to her daughter – and her partner too' – *Sunday Times*

Food Additives Erik Millstone

Eat, drink and be worried? Erik Millstone's hard-hitting book contains powerful evidence about the massive risks being taken with the health of the consumer. It takes the lid off the food we have and the food industry.

Living with Allergies Dr John McKenzie

At least 20% of the population suffer from an allergic disorder at some point in their lives and this invaluable book provides accurate and up-to-date information about the condition, where to go for help, diagnosis and cure – and what we can do to help ourselves.

Living with Stress Cary L. Cooper, Rachel D. Cooper and Lynn H. Eaker

Stress leads to more stress, and the authors of this helpful book show why low levels of stress are desirable and how best we can achieve them in today's world. Looking at those most vulnerable, they demonstrate ways of breaking the vicious circle that can ruin lives.

FOR THE BEST IN PAPERBACKS, LOOK FOR THE 🐧

PENGUIN HEALTH

Medicines: A Guide for Everybody   Peter Parish

This sixth edition of a comprehensive survey of all the medicines available over the counter or on prescription offers clear guidance for the ordinary reader as well as invaluable information for those involved in health care.

Pregnancy and Childbirth   Sheila Kitzinger

A complete and up-to-date guide to physical and emotional preparation for pregnancy – a must for all prospective parents.

The Penguin Encyclopaedia of Nutrition   John Yudkin

This book cuts through all the myths about food and diets to present the real facts clearly and simply. 'Everyone should buy one' – *Nutrition News and Notes*

The Parents' A to Z   Penelope Leach

For anyone with a child of 6 months, 6 years or 16 years, this guide to all the little problems involved in their health, growth and happiness will prove reassuring and helpful.

Jane Fonda's Workout Book

Help yourself to better looks, superb fitness and a whole new approach to health and beauty with this world-famous and fully illustrated programme of diet and exercise advice.

Alternative Medicine   Andrew Stanway

Dr Stanway provides an objective and practical guide to thirty-two alternative forms of therapy – from Acupuncture and the Alexander Technique to Macrobiotics and Yoga.

FOR THE BEST IN PAPERBACKS, LOOK FOR THE 🐧

PENGUIN HEALTH

The Prime of Your Life   Dr Miriam Stoppard

The first comprehensive, fully illustrated guide to healthy living for people aged fifty and beyond, by top medical writer and media personality, Dr Miriam Stoppard.

A Good Start   Louise Graham

Factual and practical, full of tips on providing a healthy and balanced diet for young children, *A Good Start* is essential reading for all parents.

How to Get Off Drugs   Ira Mothner and Alan Weitz

This book is a vital contribution towards combating drug addiction in Britain in the eighties. For drug abusers, their families and their friends.

Naturebirth   Danaë Brook

A pioneering work which includes suggestions on diet and health, exercises and many tips on the 'natural' way to prepare for giving birth in a joyful relaxed way.

Pregnancy   Dr Jonathan Scher and Carol Dix

Containing the most up-to-date information on pregnancy – the effects of stress, sexual intercourse, drugs, diet, late maternity and genetic disorders – this book is an invaluable and reassuring guide for prospective parents.

Care of the Dying   Richard Lamerton

It is never true that 'nothing more can be done' for the dying. This book shows us how to face death without pain, with humanity, with dignity and in peace.